FROM THE DUGOUT TO THE 19TH HOLE

My Extraordinary
Life in Sports Medicine

GREG JOHNSON

Mountain Page Press
HENDERSONVILLE, NC

Published 2021 by Mountain Page Press

ISBN: 978-1-952714-10-8
Copyright © 2021 Greg Johnson

For information, contact the publisher at:
Mountain Page Press
118 5th Ave. W.
Hendersonville, NC 28792
Visit: www.mountainpagepress.com

This is a work of creative non-fiction. All of the events in
this memoir are true to the best of the author's memory.
Some names and identifying features have been changed to
protect the identity of certain parties. The views expressed
in this memoir are solely those of the author.

The author makes reasonable efforts to present accurate
and reliable information in this book; The author is not
responsible for any errors in or omissions references or
websites listed or other information contained in this book.

CONTENTS

INTRODUCTION

When I was a kid, I did everything I could to be like my sports heros. When I played catch, I would imagine I was getting ready to field the final out of the ninth inning of the seventh game of the World Series. Or I was catching the touchdown pass that would give my team a one-point lead as time expired with the fans jumping to their feet. Every kid does that, don't they? The teams may change, the players are new every few years, and it might be a different sport, but the appeal of being a star athlete helping the hometown team win the championship—that's something every kid wants. You want big wins, great fans, and great stories!

Like pretty much everyone else, that's not what happened to me.

But I did get lucky.

I found a way to be on that field, next to the action, and help those athletes get those wins. It wasn't as glamorous as crushing a grand slam, but it was just as good. I helped a lot of people, I made a lot of friends, and I had the best seat in the house.

I was born in Superior, Wisconsin, about five hours northwest of Green Bay. We moved a couple of different times, but we finally settled in Melbourne, FL, which is even farther from Green Bay. In the late 1950s, the only way you could really get sports was either to watch it on TV or to listen to it on the radio. I had a transistor radio, and the White Sox station, WCFL, was the one that I could listen to reliably. So I would go to bed, sneak that little radio into my room, and plug in a headset. If there was a game on, I'd listen into the wee hours.

I became a Mickey Mantle fan when I was 8 years old. We were living in Alexandria, VA, and one afternoon in the early 1960s my father took me to my first game at Griffith Park in Washington, DC. The Yankees were playing the Washington Senators, but I don't remember anything about the game except for Mickey Mantle.

Radio and stadium visits got me interested in sports, but I really think that sports were just in my blood. My grandfather, Ray C. Johnson, was the athletic director, head football coach, and basketball coach at Stout State University. It's still up there, but now it's called the University of Wisconsin—Stout. He ended up as their sports guy for over thirty years.

Our family would travel up to Wisconsin every few years to spend part of our summer at our lake house in Menominee, WI. I loved those visits. My grandfather got me all the best sports equipment, and he took me to all the games. He even went to a banquet for the Green Bay Packers and brought back a Bart Starr autograph. Starr was their Hall-of-Fame quarterback. I had been interested in sports, but I got a lot more interested in the Packers. They had just won the NFL Championship game—the last one before the Super Bowl started—and they were fun to watch, so I became a Packers fan.

Introduction

My grandfather and I would talk sports whenever we had the chance. I remember talking more about baseball until I got into high school and really started to pay attention to football—both professional and collegiate. He was one of the people who supported me when I wanted to make sports my profession.

Before I could think about a profession, I had to finish high school. I wanted to play football, but I wasn't a big guy when I got to high school. I kept hoping for a growth spurt, but that never happened. I was just too small. I wanted to play baseball and football, but I just didn't have the size.

I think a lot of guys have that experience. You grow up wanting to be the next star athlete, and you might have some good hand-eye coordination or some strength or endurance, but you just stop growing. So you move on to something else. Or, in my case, you figure out another way. I knew my grandfather had a career in sports without being a player, so I had some idea of other ways to be part of a team. As I was thinking about this I met one of the guys who helped out at my high school, a guy named Joe Doller. He was a chiropractor who had worked for the Chicago Bears, and he got me interested in becoming an athletic trainer. It was Joe Doller who introduced me to the world of sports medicine.

Working with Joe meant that I could follow my dream of being involved with sports. It's easy to think of sports as all about people doing amazing things, and there's a lot of that. But there's a lot of work that nobody sees, and a lot of lessons that can help someone become a better person. I didn't know about the life lessons before I got into sports, but I learned more on the field—or at least near the field—than I learned in school. Though I want to be quick to say that I learned a lot of great stuff in school, too!

One big lesson I learned is that you have to get along with everybody on your team. The key to getting along with others is empathy. Let's take music. I was a beach guy from Florida. I liked the Beach Boys. I hated country music. I hated rap music. I would get on a bus with black guys, Latinos from across Central and South America, country rednecks, and city guys. We all needed to find a way to get along with each other or the team doesn't work. And what it makes you realize is that you've got to have some empathy for other people. I learned how to get along with just about anybody. When I learned to listen to someone else's favorite music and appreciate it, I learned to be open to all the varieties of life experience that were out in the world. I wasn't stuck, like a lot of kids are, thinking that there's just one, right way to live.

I came from the Midwest where there wasn't a lot of diversity. It was just a bunch of Swedish, Norwegian, Finnish people. When I got to Florida, I got a little bit of everything. I grew. I got exposed to other races and ethnicity and I met kids who didn't know where their next meal was coming from. I was lucky that I didn't have to worry about that, but it was only meeting other kids that I learned how lucky I was. I mean, we didn't have a lot of money, but I had clothes on my back and I had food on my table. But I had a high school teammate who lived in a bus.

Sports opened my eyes to what the real world is all about. I think sports does that for a lot of people. And I think for a kid today, looking for an opportunity to experience life and understand what it's like to share, to be a teammate, to be a team player, to understand what other people are going through in their life—sports are great for that.

Sports made me realize that there was a lot more to life than the Leave It to Beaver world in which I was raised. I'm glad that it happened because it broadened my horizons. It made me realize how much else is out there.

And sports kept me out of trouble. I never used drugs growing up. I knew guys who were OD-ing and beach bums. Because of sports I had coaches and teammates looking after me and that was great. It kept me from making some bad choices. I mean back in those days—in the early 70s—there was a lot of drug use and a lot of people doing things they weren't supposed to. I think sports kept me out of trouble because they kept me busy. I had to go to school and then practice until six o'clock, and then I had to go home and eat dinner and do homework, so between school and home I don't have a lot of time to get into trouble. On weekends I had to work. I mowed grass and worked for a moving and storage company. I don't know if my parents planned it, but they certainly weren't disappointed to see that I was a busy young man helping others and staying out of trouble.

I also learned how to listen. There's a lot of great people out there who can help you if you listen. And if we spent more 80% of our time listening and 20% of our time talking, we would all be better off because there's a lot to hear and learn. I got tips from coaches and old-timers, from teachers and mentors in sports medicine. I liked to talk a lot, but I really came to understand the value of listening.

Greg Johnson

The rest of this book is going to be me talking a lot, but a lot of these stories happened when I was listening. I had a front-row seat to some great games and some long road trips. I watched the standards of sports medicine get better each year, and I got to see up close and personal how weight training and conditioning changed my two favorite sports: baseball and golf. I had to pay my dues—over and over again—but I grew up enough to see how I could use my lessons from sports in my personal life, and that has made me a better husband and father.

ONE

WARM UPS

Every football game starts with a kickoff, every baseball season starts with a first pitch, and my journey in sports medicine started in junior high school. At Southwest Junior High School in Melbourne, FL, I was an all-around athletic trainer. I helped with the baseball, football, and basketball teams for a couple of years before moving on to the Melbourne High School.

I don't remember much about the junior high days, but high school is a little clearer. I've already mentioned Joe Doller, and it was Joe who got me thinking that sports medicine could be a career for me. Before I worked with him, I had been thinking about becoming a major league umpire. He pointed out that there aren't a lot of umps in the big leagues, but there are a lot of trainers. He helped me to see a great possibility, and he also helped me get a college scholarship. Without Joe, this book would never have been written.

I want to be clear about the work that Joe and I did. There was no sports medicine when I was in high school. At least, not like we think of it today. Back then, it was still pretty new, but I got really interested really quickly. Of course, it looked very different back then. I mean, we had Joe there, but he was just a family practice guy. He would come to the games, and he taught me the stuff that I needed to know, but it was just basic first aid stuff. It wasn't anything scientific like it is today. Back then, you just kind of learned a bit about what helped and what didn't. But we didn't have a lot of sophistication.

Take what happened when a guy "got his bell rung" in a football game. Our concussion treatment was nonexistent. We were supposed to ask some basic questions like, "What's your mother's maiden name?" That one was always my favorite. Or "How many fingers?" It feels so archaic now, but it's what we had.

Now they've got sophisticated programs. They have concussion protocols that you have to follow. A lot of guys paid a high price for our ignorance. For instance, Brett Favre said he got knocked out over 200 times during his career, and now he can't even find his way home from the grocery store. He's not that old, and I can't imagine what he's going to be like in another ten years.

I was lucky, though, that I never had anybody who had a really bad injury. Nobody died or anything like that. Anybody that we put on a stretcher board and went to the hospital was fine. We had a couple of serious injuries, but they were athletic injuries—bruises, strains, that sort of thing.

But sports medicine is more than just what happens on the playing field. Take something as basic as working out. When I started, players didn't lift weights. They thought it would be bad for their mechanics. The idea that you could help your form by working out came in the 70s. Sure a few guys here and there might lift weights, but the coaches didn't like it. Women were definitely discouraged from weight training! Then players and coaches realized that strong guys can play baseball, and everybody could play it better when they were stronger. And then everybody got bigger, stronger, faster. Coaches can help your skills on the field or the court, but a good trainer can help you lift in specific ways that are functional to the game you're playing. But all this thinking about weight training and workouts was new.

When I was looking at colleges and talking to Joe, only two schools in the country had sports medicine programs. So when I was about to graduate high school, I had to make a big decision—a decision made a lot bigger because of world events. The Vietnam War was still going on, and, when I got my draft notice, I thought I was going to Vietnam. My plan was to join the Navy because father was a Navy vet—my grandfather had been in the Army in World War I and my father in Korea, so I knew what it meant to be in the service. But I figured that if I was going to get shot, I'd rather be on a boat than in a rice paddy. It turned out that they ended the draft in December 1972, before I was old enough to qualify.

Before they ended the draft, though, I needed to make my plans. Thoughout my life, sports would be important to me in unexpected ways, and this moment was an early example. Like a lot of high school kids I didn't really know where I wanted to go to college. My high school football coach, Larry Maier, had played at the University of Tampa, and he suggested that I check them out. It was a small, private college with a small football program, but they had some big names that came out of it. One of those was a guy named Freddie Solomon who would go on to mentor Jerry Rice at the San Francisco 49ers camp. Solomon played eleven years in the NFL after being the first choice in the second round for the Miami Dolphins.

I applied to Tampa with the help of Coach Maier, and I got accepted. Coach even helped me get a partial scholarship to help with the football team. So in the fall of 1974 I headed over to Tampa, about a three-hour drive from home. I liked the school pretty well, and I worked for their head trainer, John Lopez, who was an old friend of my coach. School was interesting, and I learned a ton from Lopez, who was really my first mentor in sports medicine. Turns out that he went on to become the head trainer with the Baltimore Colts, so, while I didn't know it at the time, I was learning from one of the best. But as much as I liked the university and the work, my stay in Tampa didn't last long.

The bad news came at the end of our first season. The Tampa Bay Buccaneers were coming to town, and the school decided to drop the football program. The president of the university said "we cannot compete for fans" with the Buccaneers. So I had to look for another school.

Coach Maier came to my aid again. This time, though, he wasn't helping me from my old high school. Things change quickly in sports, and Coach Maier had been hired as the defensive coordinator at Troy State University in Troy, AL. From his new position at Troy, he arranged a scholarship for me as a trainer for the football team.

So I was off to my second school in two years.

This time, though, my experience was not so great. In fact, this was one of my worst experiences in sports.

The first weekend I was in Troy, the Ku Klux Klan held a march that went down the main street in town. I'd never seen anything like it except on TV. While the KKK rally was a problem for me, it was only one day, and they disappeared after that. The real problem for a young college student like me was that the county was dry. We had to drive all the way to Columbus, GA, to get beer. Each beer run took at least four hours.

But then it turned out that I was wrong about the rally being a one-day thing. Race was a constant issue, which I did not care for, and it hit close to home. My roommate was a black player who was dating a white woman. One day when I got back to our room, he showed me a note that had been slipped into his campus mailbox saying that he needed to stop dating the woman or he would be strung up. That was certainly a low point.

The big problem—bigger than the beer and racism—was that the team was in trouble. At the end of the 1975 season, the head coach was fired, which meant that all the other coaches had to go as well. Given all the disorder and turmoil happening, I figured it was time for me to go, too. The only good thing that came out of my experience at Troy was meeting Dr. James Andrews.

Dr. Jim Andrews—as his friends called him—was the team doctor for Troy and a surgeon at the Hughston Clinic in Columbus, GA. Dr. Andrews—along with Don Fauls at Florida

State—taught me more about sports medicine than anybody else. Dr. Andrews and I both remained part of the sports medicine world, though he gained a much greater reputation by being the person who perfected the Tommy John procedure.

I looked up to him from the first time we met, and I still consult him about major life choices. Several years after our time at Troy State, I arranged for him to help out with the Atlanta Braves, which is how he became a lifelong colleague as well as a mentor. But that's getting ahead of myself.

I knew that I had to get out of Troy, but I didn't really have a plan. So I called my old mentor, John Lopez, who was still the head trainer at the University of Tampa.

I got him on the phone one afternoon and, after quickly catching up, I said, "Doc, I got to get out of here. I just don't fit in here at all."

He said, "Well, let me make a couple of calls."

He called me back about a week later and said, "Hey, I've got some good news! I got you an opportunity to go to Florida State."

And I said, "Oh, man, but they suck." I didn't want to go there because they hadn't won a football game in two years. Then I thought for a little bit, and I said, "Well, you know what, it's a scholarship."

"Good call," John said. "Go meet Doc, Don Fauls. He's a great guy, and you'll learn a ton from him."

There's always a lot of turnover and change in sports. What I didn't know at that moment was that I wasn't the only guy heading toward Florida State after a rocky stay at a different school. A guy at the University of South Florida was leaving because they didn't have a football team, and he wanted to do football. It turned out that he was my old roommate at Tampa, Randy Oravetz, and he was also interviewing with the head student trainer at FSU.

On the day of the interview I was pretty nervous, but the conversation went really well. At the end of the day, Don Fauls had both Randy and me in the room. He said, "Guys, I know John Lopez recommended both of you, and that's good enough for me." Then he pulled something out of his desk and said, "We'd love to have you. Here's the keys to an apartment. Don't ask where it came from. Welcome to Seminole Country."

So Randy and I became roommates, again. And I was excited to get out of Troy.

When I got to Florida State for my first year, I already wasn't a fan because they had not won a football game for years. Another problem was that I wasn't an FSU fan growing up. Instead I had watched Florida football because I liked their quarterback, Steve Spurrier. But winning football games was not as important to me as being in a comfortable place, and FSU was a perfect match for me. Having Randy there was awesome as well. And I'm happy to report that we did win five games in 1976, the first year I was there.

While I was at Florida State, I worked football and base-ball, and I really got into baseball because there was a guy named Woody Woodward coaching the team. He had played shortstop for the Cincinnati Reds, and his roommate on the road had been Pete Rose. This was back in the heyday of the Big Red Machine and the really good Cincinnati Reds teams in the 70s.

I spent a good bit of time with Woodward, and we talked a lot about what it was like in Major League Baseball. After listening to his stories, I said, "Man, I want to be part of that." He told me that he knew a lot of scouts and would recommend some for me to talk to.

Woodward wasn't the only major league guy around Florida State. Dick Howser had been a player with the Yankees was the FSU first base coach for a couple of years after he retired. He had a chance to manage the Yankees for one game before he came down to FSU for a year to be the head coach for the baseball team but moved over to first base. He left to manage the Kansas City Royals for five more years after that. Florida State was a great place to learn about baseball and make some important connections.

For me the late 70s at FSU were taken up by a full schedule of classes and work at Tully Gym, which housed the training room. I worked for football and baseball, mostly, but I also worked with basketball, track, and all the women's sports. I was so busy with school and work that I dated very little, but I want to say a few things two women who taught me about real life.

The first woman was an athletic trainer who I met while working at Tully. She was bright, bubbly, and beautiful. She was also Jewish. The Jewish part is important because it was the issue that eventually broke us up. We dated throughout the fall quarter, and when Thanksgiving break came around I asked if I could visit her during the holiday. It's a pretty safe holiday, I thought. Lots of family to keep everyone distracted and no gifts to get judged on. When she said no, I was shocked and hurt. I asked her why, and she admitted that her Jewish family would not accept a non-Jew. I was devastated. It was my first experience with real heartbreak.

It wasn't long before I had the chance to learn another important lesson. I had to take some biology and physiology classes at another local school, Florida A&M, which was—and still is—an outstanding HBCU (Historically Black Colleges and Universities). The classes were a little outside my major, but I knew that taking these courses would help with my career as an athletic trainer. Early in the quarter I was heading to an applied anatomy class, but I got completely lost. I was wandering the hallways of a huge building when I felt a tap on my shoulder, and heard a woman ask, "Are you lost?" I turned around to see a beautiful African-American woman looking at me. I told her that I was, that I was looking for the applied anatomy class. She pointed and said, "The white school is over yonder."

I stammered for a moment before she started laughing and said that her friends had put her up to it.

It turned out that she was going to the same class, so we walked to the room together.

We became friends and study mates. After about six weeks of spending a lot of time together, she asked, "Why haven't you made a pass at me? Is it because I'm black?"

It sort of surprised me. She was so beautiful, I had assumed she was just out of my league. But I knew I couldn't say that, so I said, "No, it's not that. I just didn't think you'd be interested in me." Come to find out she was interested, and I was definitely interested, so for the next three months we had a great time together. I could hardly believe that this amazing woman wanted to spend so much extracurricular time with me. We were doing well together, but when it came time for me to meet her family it all sort of stalled. She had a lot of excuses as to why I couldn't meet them. One day before fall break, I point-blank asked her why. She said that her parents didn'tt know she was dating a white guy, and she hadn't told them because she knew they wouldn't approve. I don't know whether her coming from Mississippi made a difference, but I think it did. Things cooled off pretty quickly after that. But that moment taught me a lot about race.

Florida is a great place to heal your heartache, though. The state brings all kinds of people from all over to relax and recuperate, including celebrities and sports stars. I met Johnny Unitas in 1974 while at a bar that I frequented in Melbourne Beach. He had just retired and was in his early 40s. I think I was the only one to recognize him when he came in. I went over to where he was sitting and spoke with him. I told him how much I enjoyed watching him play, and he was nice to me. We sat and talked football for a few hours, and I really appreciated his generosity.

Also in 1974, John Lopez, still the head athletic trainer at Tampa, invited Randy and me to work the Tangerine Bowl in Orlando as part of his staff. This was my first real exposure to a national TV audience and big-time college football. I was on the sidelines for the largest crowd I had ever seen, and I was thrilled. While I would never work much in football, I loved the excitement that those fans brought to the games.

After graduating in 1978, I was accepted into graduate school, which shocked everyone in my family. Here's a kid that no one thought would even get into college becoming the first person in my immediate family to go to graduate school. My motivation for going was twofold: First, I wanted to prove not only that everyone was wrong that I could not make it through college but also that I could go to graduate school and succeed. Second, I wanted to continue my work in sports medicine as a graduate assistant athletic trainer. Getting that master's degree diploma in my hands in 1980 was something that, to this day, I am very proud of. The bachelor's degree I received was for all those that said I wasn't college material in 1973; the master's was for me. In fact, I had an opportunity to go back and get a PhD, but I said no. I had had enough of studying and was more interested in working winter ball for the Braves in then I was in going back to school.

By the fall of 1978 I was working full-time as a trainer, going to grad school full-time for two quarters and, in the spring and summer, working for the Atlanta Braves. During the grad school years I lived off campus with Randy Oravetz in a one-bedroom apartment. Life—and my schedule—was full, but there was not much time for a personal life or dating, even if I experienced a lot of joy and fulfillment in other parts of my life. Toward the end of my degree program, I began thinking about beginning a new life after school, a life that hopefully included moving into a full-time job with the Braves.

Grad school went pretty quickly, so in the winter of 1981 my full-time work in the sports world began. And now I was free to pursue my career. It was the beginning of an amazing ride in several professional sports leagues that would last for more than a decade.

TWO

ON DECK

Before I could move into the professional ranks, I needed to develop my connections a bit more. I started working on that before grad school. It was when I was getting toward the end of my time at college that I asked Doc Fauls if he could help me find a position after I graduated. He must have been working hard for me because one day in early 1978 Doc called me into his office and said he might have something for me with the Braves. Doc and Woody Woodward had a connection with the Atlanta organization, Paul Snyder, the director of scouting for Atlanta.

When I met with Snyder, he said, "You know, it's not all glamour. You're going to have to start out in the minor leagues somewhere, and it's going to be hard work."

I said, "Well, I'd love the opportunity."

He liked that answer. "Let me bring it up to the VP of minor league operations, and we'll see where it goes."

I said, "Okay, fine." I gave him my number, and I just had to wait.

And then one of the most embarrassing moments of my life happened.

I got a call about a week later. I picked up, and I heard a voice on the phone that said, "This is Henry Aaron."

I said, "Yeah, right. Get outta here." And I hung up.

The phone rang again. "This is Henry Aaron," said the voice. And I hung up again.

I thought it was my buddies playing a joke on me, and I didn't think anything about it until I got another call.

This time, a woman's voice said, "This is Susan Bailey with the Atlanta Braves." She said, "Please don't hang up."

"Oh," I said. "I see." And I paused, then said, "Was that...?"

"Yes, it was."

"Okay."

It turns out that Susan Bailey was Henry Aaron's executive assistant, and I guess they figured that I wouldn't hang up on a woman.

Aaron finally got on the phone and said, "Hey, we'd like to talk to you. Can you come up to Atlanta?"

Of course I said that I would. He told me that they would send a plane ticket so that I could fly up for the job interview.

You know, I got on that plane, went to the team offices, and I got the job. I almost couldn't sleep that night, I was so excited to be working in baseball. But Paul Snyder was right. It wasn't going to be all glamour. My first job in baseball was in Greenwood, South Carolina. I had no idea where Greenwood was, nor did I really care. They had the right name though—the Braves—even if it was their low minor league team, single-A.

14

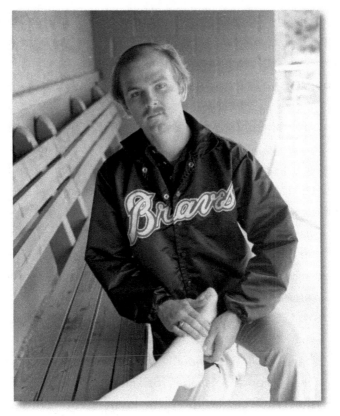

Greg working for the Braves

I made $4,700 a year, which was low even in the 70s. The job was from spring training in February until the season ended in September. But I was thrilled. I mean, to get a job like that meant the world to me, and an opportunity like that doesn't come along every day.

I hate to say it, but my first impression of Hank Aaron wasn't much. He couldn't remember my name, nor where I was working while I attended my first spring training in 1978. Hank had a problem remembering player and staff names throughout my career with the Braves. But it was an honor and a thrill to work with him, and I got to know him pretty well over the next several years. And my impression got better the more time I spent with him.

I moved up to Greenwood before spring training and rented an apartment for $60 a month. It was above the landlady's garage and had no air conditioning or insulation. That first year I saved $3,000 out of my $4,700 salary by renting that cheap apartment and eating in the locker room and on the road and letting the club pay for it.

I was still in grad school at the time. So I went to work for the Braves from February until September, and from September until February I went back to Florida State as a grad assistant for the fall quarter. I kept that schedule from 1978 to 1980 as I was working on getting my master's degree. As I said before, it was a busy few years.

When I was in Greenwood, I was everything for that team. I was the equipment manager, road manager, traveling secretary, shoe shine guy, laundry dude, locker room maintenance man—you name it, I did it. I even drove the old school bus that was our transportation for away games. But that wasn't all. I was still trying to make ends meet, which meant finding ways to improve my cash flow. One way I made a little extra money was stocking the Coke machine in the locker room. That doesn't sound like a way to make extra cash, but what you could do was get the guy from the Coke distributor to set the price a little higher on the machine and then keep the dime or so difference between what you owed the distributor and the money that actually came in. I also sold t-shirts and batting gloves—equipment and gear that the players didn't get as part of the uniform—to the guys.

That's part of the game that fans don't see. They don't see what these players and people in the business go through to get where they want to go, which is the big leagues. And it was tough—we all had a lot of dues to pay. But another thing a lot of people don't see is you always had someone who would be willing to teach you whatever you needed to learn—on-field or life skills. Basically, if you're willing to listen and learn, you'll find mentors everywhere, and that's one of the great things about sports. And it makes the dues a little easier to pay.

For example, I learned how to get that extra cash from listening to older guys in AA spring training. I think most baseball fans know that all the teams gather in either Arizona or Florida. We went to spring training in West Palm Beach, but what you might now know if you don't hang around during spring training is that maybe a half dozen different minor league teams will be sequestered near you, so you had a lot of chances to talk to players and staff from across the leage. The major league teams would also be nearby, but in a lot nicer, better places. In the minor leagues you're putting in a lot of hours, you're learning your trade, and you have guys who show you how it works. For me, the most important guy was Sam Ayoub.

Being near the big league players during spring break also made you want it more. You could see over the fence and watch guys like Dale Murphy and Phil Niekro and Chris Chambliss, and you'd think, 'God, I want to get there someday.' But that takes so much talent and work that only a few make it. So you pay your dues, you listen to your mentors, and you work hard.

One of the first people I met in the spring of 1978 was Ted Turner. Bobby Cox introduced him to me in the dugout of the Braves spring training site. I shook his hand and said, "Nice to meet you Mr. Turner."

Turner replied, "Ted's my name, and baseball's my game."

In those years Ted was very active with the Braves, and it was pretty common to see him around spring training or at home games. Everything Ted touched seemed to turn to gold. He bought a money-losing TV station in Atlanta and turned it into the Superstation in just a few years. I remember him talking in the dressing room about starting a twenty-four-hour news station, and nobody thought anybody would want to watch the news for twenty-four hours. I guess that's why he's one of the wealthiest men in America and I'm not.

I worked with a lot of guys who weren't as wealthy as Ted Turner. Alan "Dirty Al" Gallagher was the first manager that I worked for in Greenwood, SC, and he was a real piece of work. Like his name suggests, he was a dirty guy—I mean, physically dirty. He didn't want his uniform washed, so that was always dirty. And we were playing games all over the South, so it got to smelling real bad real quick. Gallagher was a gruff guy, but a really good guy. He also worked hard to help the young players in the minor leagues. Even as manager he was willing to help guys with their fielding techniques, but he also took an interest in the players' careers and preparing for life outside baseball. I remember him helping more than a couple guys think about how to deal with the money they were earning.

And he was always willing to tell stories. Minor league guys tended to gravitate to the former major leaguers to hear the stories.

Dirty Al and Bob Veale, our pitching coach, taught me a lot about the game of baseball in my first year in the business. Both guys were great at talking about how the game should be played and telling us about the golden years of baseball with players like Willie McCovey, Roberto Clemente, Willie Mays, and Mickey Mantle. They missed the days when baseball was a rougher sport. They told stories about guys sliding spikes-first into second-basemen and leading with shoulders into catchers when they crossed home plate. But a lot of times the rough stuff was all about getting your team-mate's back and making sure the team could win.

During my entire time with the Braves organization, Hank Aaron was my boss. He was the Director of Minor League Operations, which meant he was the boss for a lot guys.

One of my memorable dealings with Hank was in 1979. It was spring training, and I was mostly sitting on the

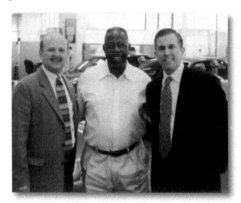

Greg with Hank Aaron

sidelines because I had broken my hand. Since I wasn't doing as much as the other trainers, Hank invited me to go out and have drinks with him and other Braves administrative staff at the major league hotel, the Hyatt in West Palm Beach. Hank never wanted to drink and drive, so he asked me to drive him around in the station wagon a local dealership had loaned him to drive during spring training. We got into the station wagon to head over from the Day's Inn to the Hyatt—the difference between the minor leagues and the Bigs.

In the car he handed me a roll of cash and asked me to peel off $100. He said, "Greg, no matter what, don't give me any more." Hank had a tendency to spend more freely while drinking. I later counted the roll without him knowing, and he was carrying around $5,000 with him.

So off we headed to the Hyatt. We met general manager Bill Lucas, manager Bobby Cox, Hank's brother, Tommie Aaron, and after a few minutes, Ted Turner. After several hours of some pretty heavy drinking and Hank not speaking very well because of the liquor, Bill Lucas, who was Hank's brother-in-law, turned to everyone and said, "I sure hope Hank's not driving."

I spoke up, "I'm the driver."

At the end of the evening I got Hank into the car, and he turned to me and said, "Greg, let's go to Ft. Lauderdale and get some conch salad." Hank loved to get conch salad during spring training.

I said, "Hank, it's late. We should get back to the hotel and get some sleep."

On Deck

Hank insisted on going, but I stayed firm and told him that we weren't going, that I was going to drive us to the hotel. When we arrived, I had a hard time getting Hank up to his second-floor room. When we got to the room, he sort of slid down the wall to the floor, and I had to fumble through his pants pockets to find his key. Right about this time a couple of people walked by, and I was sure they wondered if I was robbing the guy.

I finally got the door open, helped Hank up, got him inside, and over to his bed—and all this with one broken hand. Just as I got all 200 pounds of him to the bed, he got sick. At that point, I was done. So I just pushed him over on his bed and left.

The next morning, Hank came into the training room at the Braves spring training site and asked, "Greg, did I give you my money last night?" I said "Yes," pulled out the roll of $5,000, and flipped it to him. Without counting it, he said "Thanks" and put it away. He was a very trusting guy. I had never seen that much money in my life! That's more than what I made my first year with the Braves.

I soon became Hank's driver and golf mate during spring training. One golf outing, which was our last, was especially memorable. An executive, nine-hole course was right next to our spring training facility, and one day Hank asked me to go with him to play while the rest of the minor leaguers were on the road playing the Yankees in Ft. Lauderdale. At one hole, Hank teed off and, as soon as he hit his tee shot, out from the woods came two guys in a golf cart. Neither of us saw them while teeing off, but the ball was in the air and it seemed to have radar-lock on the two golfers. We both yelled "Fore!" Sure enough, the ball hit one of the passengers, and he fell out of the cart. Hank and I raced down to them, and Hank said, "Shit, Greg, I hope I didn't kill the guy!"

We got there and saw that the guy was ok, but he was still laying on the ground. He looked up and said, "Hey, aren't you Hank Aaron?"

Hank said, "Yes, I am."

At that point the guy only wanted an autograph and Hank gladly gave him one. That's the last time Hank played golf, as far as I know. He turned his athletic attention to tennis.

Hank always had good people around him, and that included Bill Lucas, the general manager of the Atlanta Braves when I was hired in 1978. In fact, he signed my first contract. Bill was one of the nicest men I ever met in baseball. He remembered everyone and knew their name—unlike Hank. And he was Hank's brother-in-law, so I guess the Braves must have really felt like family for Hank.

Lucas was the first black GM in Major League Baseball, and it was a true honor to work with him. He died soon after I was hired, and it was terrible to see such a talented man get taken so young.

From the beginning, I tried to be as useful as I could for everyone with the Braves because you never know when the next opportunity will show up, and I wanted to be ready for anything that came my way. At one of my first spring training camps, Hank Aaron told me that all the minor league ballplayers needed to have physicals before the season, but the Braves usual doctors in Atlanta didn't have the staff for it.

The medical practice had enough resources to deal with the big league club, but not the minor league guys. Hank was asking around to see if any of the guys on the training staff knew anybody.

I immediately thought of my mentor, Dr. Jim Andrews, so I said that I knew a great guy at the Hughston Clinic who might be interested.

"Can you get in touch with him?" Hank said.

"I'll call him today."

When I reached Dr. Andrews and explained the situation, he said that he'd be happy to help. A few days later Dr. Andrews showed up with a bunch of people from the clinic, including Tad Blackburn and Pat Jones. I think he just pulled everyone who would fit in the company's private King Air plane.

Over the course of three days, Dr. Andrews and his colleagues took care of all the physicals. I couldn't believe how hard they worked to get that job done. At the end of the third day, Hank and I drove them back to the airport. As we were loading up their luggage, Hank took Dr. Andrews aside and said, "Ok, Doc, what's the damage?"

Dr. Andrews pulled out a fairly thick business envelope and handed it over without a word. Hank nodded, and we watched them close up the King Air.

As the plane started to pull away, Hank opened the envelope and started to laugh. I asked him what was so funny, and he held up three blank pages.

"He's my man. No doubt about that," Hank said, still chuckling.

That's just the kind of personality that Jim Andrews had. And that was one of his very first gigs with professional sports.

I'm proud of the fact that I connected Jim Andrews with the Braves, though I got a bit of political pushback for doing it. Andrews worked himself up the ladder with the Braves, which is not surprising at all. The minor leagues were full of guys who were either climbing the ladder, or heading back down. One of my favorites was Leo Mazzone.

Leo was a former major league pitcher who had a short run with the San Francisco Giants. He was a pitching coach in Greenwood, and even then he was doing the in-game rocking motion that became his signature for years with Atlanta and, briefly, Baltimore.

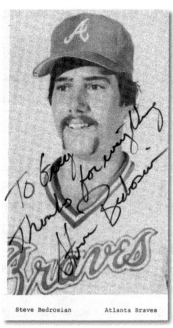

Steve Bedrosian   Atlanta Braves

Steve Bedrosian

Mazzone was a fiery competitor. I remember that we had some great up-and-coming pitchers, guys like Steve Bedrosian (the National League Cy Young Winner in 1982), Craig McMurtry, Jim Acker, and Ken Dayley. One particular week stands out. None of them were pitching well, and they all got bombed. Leo got all fired up and said, "What kind of dumbass drafted these guys!" But they all recovered and went on to have great careers.

24

Leo was a great pitching coach, but he could get mad at the drop of a hat.

We had some great, long bus rides together in the five or more years Leo and I spent in the minor leagues. On one of those rides, Leo told me about not being fateful in a relationship: "You can do anything except have intercourse and still be faithful." I was never sure about that, and his wife—a beautiful woman named Gregg (with two g's!)—was definitely not sure. They didn't stay together all that long.

I can say one more thing about Leo—his coaching was fueled by beer. One year Leo figured out that from the start of spring training in February to the end of the minor league season in September he drank about 2,500 beers. At the end of the season, he would always quit and not have another beer until spring training the next season.

Leo wasn't the only one who came to work thirsty. Beer was a constant in baseball, but the training staff had more, stranger things to deal with than the occasional hangover. One day in spring training some of the players were complaining about bad cases of athlete's foot. I mentioned it to Luke Appling, who had been around baseball since the 30s, and he told me to tell them all to pee on their feet. I looked at him, but he wasn't smiling. I said, "Are you kidding?" Luke just shrugged and said it was the best remedy for athlete's foot. He'd been around for so long, and seen so many things on the field and in the locker room, that I believed him. I don't know how all the players treated themselves, but they did it. And guess what? It worked!

We all called Luke "Old Aches and Pains," and he was one of the most interesting, funny guys in the old guard of baseball. Luke was a great shortstop with the Chicago White Sox in the 30s and 40s, and was one of the very few players to play for twenty seasons. When I met him, Luke had been a hitting instructor for most of the 70s. He'd continue that work into the 80s.

Luke use to say that the "kids" of the day didn't have the work habits of the "old-timers." He certainly hadn't let his work habits slip, and he kept himself in good shape for a guy in his 60s. But he did have one very definite weird attitude: Luke hated having his uniform—or anything else—washed. Old Aches and Pains and Dirty Al were kind of like brothers that way.

Luke was one of my favorite coaches, and he was a great ambassador for baseball. During breaks and on road trips I would sit for hours and listen to Luke tell stories about the old days. We'd be just about done for the day, and he'd say, "Stick with me kid, and I'll tell you how we used to do it." He told me stories of Bob Feller, Ted Williams, Joe DiMaggio, and all the stars of the golden days of baseball.

I always wanted to hear about baseball history, and there were always guys around ready to tell their stories, just like Luke. Clete Boyer was another one. He was a hitting instructor in the minor league organization of the Braves in the late 70s and 80s. Clete was probably the second-best third basemen in the American League during his time in the 60s. The only one better was Brooks Robinson who played with the Baltimore Orioles. Clete had a brother named Cloyd who was a pitching coach with the Braves. Clete and I used to hang out and go through several beers together during my first year in Greenwood. He knew I was a Yankee fan—specifically a Mickey Mantle fan—as a kid. Clete also talked about Joe Pepitone, who was the first guy he ever saw with a hair dryer in the locker room. He told us stories about winning the World Series with the Yankees. All of us listened with a keen ear, because most of us had never experienced anything like that. It was a dream come true to hear first-hand what that experience was like. Some of my favorite stories were the ones he told about Yogi Berra, the great Yankees catcher who had quirky sayings like, "Baseball is 90% physical and 15% mental."

Clete was also the guy who actually made one of my dreams come true. He came to me one day, and he said, "Hey, aren't we going to play the Pittsburgh Pirates team in Charleston?"

I said, "Yeah."

"Well, Mickey Mantle is going to be in town. You want to go to dinner with us?"

"Are you kidding?" I said.

Clete knew that I'd started a scrapbook on Mantle back in 1962, when I was ten. By the late 70s it was several hundred pages long, and I really wanted to give the whole book to him. It had been a dream of mine for years at that point.

I don't remember much about that Charleston game, but afterward we went to dinner. We pulled up at this nice steakhouse, and I was just nervous as hell. You don't usually get the opportunity to meet a hero and fulfill a dream. People had been telling me for years, "Oh, you'll never meet Mickey. Why do you keep that scrapbook? You'll never get a chance to give it to him." But I never lost faith that I'd meet him. And that day was the day.

We walked in, and there he was. I tried to be cook, but I was having trouble even talking. Mickey was great though, so we ordered food, drank a bunch of beers, and it all started to feel pretty good. He even called me "Doc" the whole evening. The strange thing is that this dinner with Mickey was the highlight of my professional career, even though it had nothing to do with anything on the field.

I remember that I asked him about injuries. I was the team trainer, so I was always interested in stuff like that. I said, "You had a lot of injuries in your career. How did that affect your career?"

He said, "You know, I never thought I was going to live to be the age of 50."

"Why?"

He told me that every male Mantle up to that point died right before the age of 50.

"What happened?"

"They all had black lung disease from working in coal mines. I thought I was just going to die young, so I was going to have a good time." That answer told me a lot about his choices—and reputation—off the field. It made sense to me at the time, but I know he came to regret those choices. I still wonder what his career would have been like if he had made different ones.

We got to the end of dinner, and I started to get fidgety, thinking about the scrapbook. Eventually I brought it out and handed it over to him. He took it and looked at it for a while, then he said, "Nah, I don't want to keep this."

I was a little surprised, but I said, "I wish you would."

"Well," he said, "That's great, Doc. Ok."

We talked a while longer, and he signed a ball that I still have today. He wrote, "Thanks, Doc. Best wishes."

I treasure that ball, but the bad news is that I had fourteen of his baseball cards in that scrapbook. They're worth well over $10,000 today. But you know what? It was worth it. Because I said when I was ten years old that I wanted to do this thing, and who gets a chance to make a promise to themselves at that age and actually see it through?

I went back to Greenwood feeling pretty good, but my conversation that night stayed with me.

Professional success for any athlete is partly skill and partly physical conditioning.

After several years as a student and a young professional, I started noticing which of the players were working out. Jim Bouton was one of them. Bouton was a great pitcher and the controversial author of Ball Four, a book about a year in the majors. He had been mostly out of baseball for a while when Ted Turner sent him an invitation to training camp in 1978. A lot of times, the minor leagues would have guys rehabilitating injuries or otherwise trying to make it back to the Show. Unlike a lot of them, Jim would actually make it, but not for long. Still, it was a thrill to meet Jim. He had been a twenty-game winner with the Yankees in the 60s, and he was cool to meet and talk with about the old days with them. During long bus rides, he would tell me stories about Mickey Mantle and how he was as a teammate. I would hear more about Mantle over my years with the Braves, but Jim was the first guy to share those stories with me.

Baseball is full of stories, but it also has its reliable cycles. After we closed everything down in the fall, we only had to wait a little while—about four months—for spring training. And spring training with the Braves meant that we were often placed near the Yankees in Ft. Lauderdale, which was great for me because it meant that I could almost always see my favorite team practicing.

In 1981, I remember being at the Yankees field watching a pregame warmup. George Steinbrenner was walking around the batting cage and decided that the Yankee batting helmets were too dirty for his liking. He went off on the equipment manager, yelling about how the helmets made the team look bad. Steinbrenner told the bat boys to take all the helmets into the clubhouse to clean them. With all the helmets gone, batting practice had to stop, so the whole day got behind schedule—even the game was delayed. Steinbrenner was a perfectionist, and maybe that's why the Yankees were so good during his time with the team. But I still feel bad for the equipment guy and the bat boys.

Sports seems pretty straightforward from the outside. You yell at the batboys (or you don't). You practice. You play the games. You draft new guys and start practicing again. But it's a complicated business, and the real goal of winning is to get fans in the seats. That's easy for clubs like the Yankees and Braves, but it's a lot harder for the minor league teams. So the owners try a lot of things to make a visit to the park worth it. Sometimes they put in playgrounds and other family-friendly spaces, and other times they brought in Max Patkin, the Clown Prince of Baseball. I first saw Max perform during my time with the Greenwood club. He was quite a sight! Patkin would throw dirt at the umpires, wear a filthy, ragged uniform that looked like he had worn it every day for the last thirty years. And if you thought a coach would cuss, they had nothing on Max. He would use the foulest language during his gigs. He could make a boring game a lot of fun.

But I didn't just see him on the field. He would frequently join us after the games in the hotel bar and hang out with us for several rounds of drinks. Max always had great stories about the different parks he appeared in during his career. Even with all the beautiful, new parks out there, I still miss the wild fun of Max Patkin.

There were a lot of guys like Patkin, guys who had a career that kept them in the game but not actually on the field. And there are a lot of guys who spend a lot of time in the dugout. Brian Snitker and I were on several minor league teams during my time with the Braves. His career was ok, but as a friend and a person he was fabulous. He was destined to become a great coach even during his playing career in the minor leagues. He went on to have a long career and is still a coach in the Braves system. At the time when I'm writing, he is the manager of the Atlanta Braves and won Manager of the Year in 2018.

I don't mean to brag, but I had a good start to my career in baseball. In 1980 I was selected as the East All Star team trainer for the Southern League. This was a great honor because the coaches selected you, which meant that they had noticed and valued my work, and it felt very good to have that attention early on. The game itself was played in

Memphis, TN, on the only astroturf field in the league. The team was full of players who ended up in the Show, but the biggest name was a future Yankee star named Don Mattingly. We all knew at the time he was going to become a major league player and a star.

All that travel, the routines of the road, all of that can really get to you and start to take a toll. It didn't take long for me to see that a lot of the physical stuff wasn't really physical at all. A lot of sports stuff is in the head. I could help a guy with icing a shoulder or doing hamstring stretches, but sometimes it's just listening, and I learned that I had to be like a psychiatrist. And it wasn't just about stuff on the field.

There was a lot of family stuff, too. In baseball, we were on the road every week, and when we weren't on the road, we had a game almost every day, and those could go until eleven o'clock at night. After the game, what do you do? You go home and go to bed, but it's real late at night. And then the next day you have to be at the ballpark in the afternoon for a night game again. If you have position drills or the coach wants you for something, you might have to be in earlier, so you don't have a whole lot of time to spend with your family.

For most of us, our teammates became our family, including all the medical people and the coaches. Those relationships can get pretty deep, and that's the biggest piece that I miss. So I learned to work with the players like they were family, and I tried to help them get their heads in the right space as well as patching up their bodies.

Those days and weeks away from wives and kids is another kind of dues we all had to pay. For me, that meant two divorces.

Being on the road all the time is not very conducive to marriage. Marriage is hard enough as it is. I keep hearing that around fifty percent of marriages in the US end up in divorce. In sports it has to be ten points higher than that.

I should have seen it coming in my first marriage. She knew I was in baseball, but she wasn't much of a fan. I tried to explain it to her. I said, "Listen, this is what I do for a living. It's long days and a lot of travel, and I hope you understand."

Within two weeks after the wedding I was in spring training. She called me up one night, just crying really hard. Sobbing. She was lonely. She said, "Where are you? We just got married, and I never see you!"

That was a rough moment. I said, "Hun, please. This is what I told you it was going to be like."

So it became a real issue.

And then, within a year and a half, we were divorced. She gave me an ultimatum one day. She said, "You need to make a choice. You chose me, and now you need to choose me again. It's either me or the highway."

I said, "I'm not gonna be threatened with ultimatums. This is what I told you. This is my job. This is my career."

So that one didn't work out. The second marriage was years later, after I left professional sports, but I was still working with college athletes, the PGA Tour, and other teams for extra money and to keep my practice sharp. I also watched sports to relax. But that's a story for another time.

THREE

RUNNING THE BASES

B y the end of my time in Greenwood, I was learning that the biggest issue in professional baseball was alcohol, not drugs. Were there drugs? Yes, sure. But the biggest struggles I saw were with alcohol. It's cheap and easily available. It doesn't give you an edge in a game, but it takes the edge off after a game. Sadly, a lot of guys would take it way too far.

I've never used drugs in my life. I was too scared. I was always afraid that using drugs would cost me something. I had coaches and mentors who looked after me, and they read me the riot act when I stepped out of line. And I'm glad they did. They were like father figures, and I always managed to get straightened out.

But it's also easy not to listen. Sports offers a lot of lessons, and I've tried to pay attention to those lessons over the years. It's easy when it's someone like Jim Andrews or Don Fauls, but it can be just as easy to ignore them, especially when you have a lot of other people around you telling you how great you are. I'm not saying I'm particularly special, and

I've made a lot of mistakes, but I'm grateful for mentors who got my attention, and I'm glad that I had the sense to listen. It breaks my heart to see young guys get bad advice—or not listen to the good advice—and have to spend the rest of their lives finding their way back to themselves and their families.

I found those mentors at each step of my career. High school, college, Greenwood. My stay at Greenwood didn't last long, though, and so, like so many others working in sports, I had to move on. This time the move wasn't far, just down the road to Savannah to join the double-A club there. So at least I was moving up!

Our road trips for Greenwood were in a big school bus, and Savannah was no different. These trips weren't always short ones, either, like to other towns in North and South Carolina. We were all over the South—Florida, Alabama, and all over—and we started judging the length of road trips by how much beer it would take to get there. You might have a six-pack trip or a twelve-pack trip, and we would make sure we all knew how long the trip was going to be because we had to bring our own. You also had to bring your own cooler, though the team would usually gave you with a sandwich and chips. So we'd line up with our coolers, grab some food, and throw that in on top of the beer before loading up on the bus.

One of the other teams in our league was way over in Memphis, and I remember one trip we had in particular. The trip started late at night after a game. We were all tired, but we'd also started into the beer as we headed down the road.

Something to keep in mind is that there's a hierarchy of seating. I don't know if everyone does this, but our seating arrangement was something like this: the manager sat in the front left seat, the pitching coach sat in the front right seat, the trainer (that would be me) sat in the front second left seat, the other coach sat in the second right seat, and so on. The guys up front got to sit by themselves, but the players had to share their seats.

On this trip, we had Eddie Haas, Bobby Dews, and Leo Mazzone up front—and those guys could put away a lot of beer. We had been a while on the road, and Eddie finally needed to get to the pisser in the back of the bus. The only way to do that was to climb over a few seats because a lot of guys had fallen asleep, and they relaxed quite a bit, so legs and feet were like a fishing net down the aisle. Eddie decided that the way to get past this obstacle was to climb to the top of the seats and somehow walk on the tops of the seats all the way to the back. We all thought this was not a good idea. Trying to pull off something like that when he was stone, cold sober and the bus was stopped would have been difficult, and neither of those two things was true at the moment. But we couldn't change his mind, so he set off. He made it over a couple of seats, which was impressive, but then the inevitable happened and gravity grabbed him. It looked like he was going to be ok, but then he held up his foot. And a sandwich. Which he was wearing like a shoe. Turns out that one of our pitchers, Tim Cole, had bought one of those cheap, styrofoam coolers, and Eddie had managed to break the cooler and shove his foot into Tim's dinner.

Not all road trips had that kind of hilarity, but we did have some good times on the bus. And sometimes off the bus.

Greg Johnson

The trip to Memphis happened several times in a season, and we sometimes had to do a long road swing from there down to Florida. While the bus was mostly reliable, we could run into trouble. One incident always comes to mind.

Our bus broke down somewhere in rural Mississippi early in the morning. We were in the middle of nowhere. It was four or five in the morning, and it was already hot as hell, so nobody wanted to stay on a bus with no air conditioning. We all got out and looked around, and all that was around was a field with a bunch of cattle. I mean, it was nowhere. Eddie told everyone to stay close to the bus.

Well, one of our pitchers didn't listen. Steve Bedrosian, who ended up winning the Cy Young, looked out into the field and saw this big bull. A couple of other guys saw it, too, and they started telling Bedrosian that he could take this bull. I don't know what the hell they were yelling, but he decided that he would go into the field and challenge that bull.

Bedrosian climbed the fence, and started to walk over to the bull. At first, nothing happened, but the guys back at the bus kept egging him on. So he kept walking toward it. But the bull didn't react. So he started yelling at the bull, and that set the animal off. And those things are fast! Bedrosian ran faster than I had ever seen him go, and he got to the fence near us, but he got hung up in the barbed wire. He was struggling to get over to the other side, and all of us were just dying with laughter, except for Eddie Haas, who saw what was happening and helped Bedrosian over the fence just in time.

While I was there to witness Bedrosian take on the bull, I can't verify what happened on the occasion of this incident with Matt Sinatro. He was a funny, goofy guy, who we all liked. Once, when we were on one of our several road trips in the minor leagues, he came into the clubhouse and told a story that's never been topped in my entire career with the Braves.

A lot of the guys would find dates on road trips, which sometimes had negative consequences for players—and managers—with wives and girlfriends at home. On this particular afternoon, Sinatro was in the locker room with a bunch of us, and he said he had picked up a woman at a local bar, and they had gone back to her house. When they totally into it, and they were about to take the final step, the woman said, "If you are not going to call me after this, then don't continue." He then said the funniest thing any of us had ever heard, "Ok, I won't." Then he told us that he got up, put his clothes on, and left. The other ball players in the locker room laughed so hard they were rolling on the floor. He didn't stop hearing about that for a long time.

But Matt just had a different attitude.

With a lot of ballplayers, they have some great skills, but aren't well-rounded enough to stay in the league. Matt Sinatro was like that—an excellent defensive catcher, but his offensive numbers were never good. Still, he went on to have a pretty good career as a coach.

It's easy to forget how bad the road trips were when you have moments like those with Bedrosian and Sinatro, and I still miss those times. There's an intense bonding that happens, and you learn to rely on your teammates for craziness and help. It's still a business, though, and as fun as sports can be, it can also leave you feeling pretty bad when the guys you've been hanging out with get traded or cut.

The higher ups didn't always know the team as well as they thought. Hank Aaron, as I've mentioned, had a problem remembering ball players names. One day the phone rang in the training room, and I answered it, and it was Hank (I had learned to recognize his voice by this point). He asked for our manager, Eddie Haas, and I told Hank that he was at batting practice. He told me to give Eddie a message that we needed to release Steve Bedrosian, one of our better pitchers. Knowing Hank's tendency to get players' names wrong, I said, "Hank, I think you've got the wrong player."

Without hesitating, he said, "I'll call you back."

A few minutes later the phone rang again and it was Susan Bailey, Hank's trusted executive assistant for over twenty years. She told me to leave Bedrosian alone and gave me another name to hand over to Eddie.

I spent a lot of time with Hank during my career with the Braves, and I came to know him as a fair and caring person. He wanted to help ball players, but he could not understand why they had such a hard time playing a game that came so naturally to a superstar like him. I remember one spring training when this point really hit home. I was standing near Hank and Hall-of-Fame-pitcher Bob Gibson around the batting cage, watching guys work on their mechanics.

Hank said, "I don't understand why hitting is so hard for these kids."

Gibson replied, "Hell, Hank, I can't understand why painting the black with a pitch is so hard."

One of my last memories of spending time with Hank was at the premiere of his movie, Hank Aaron: Chasing the Dream. The film documented Hank's pursuit of Babe Ruth's homerun record. That was a very difficult year for Hank. Throughout the season he was called racist names, had his life threatened, and spent a lot of time living in fear in the locker room. After the film, Hank turned to me and asked, "Greg, what did you think?"

That was one of the toughest moments of my life. I told Hank that I was embarrassed to be white after seeing how whites treated Hank.

Hank smiled and said, "Greg, those people are not you. You got nothing to worry about."

I had learned in my life that sports meant that you meet all kinds of people, which helped me—and it helps others, too, I think—develop empathy and understanding. I saw both in Hank Aaron that day. And it hurt me to see that so many others who shared my love of sports hadn't been able to develop their own empathy and understanding. It goes to show that listening and learning are hard, but they make us better people.

The last time I spent meaningful time with Hank was on a trip to speak at the Baseball Academy meeting in Birmingham at the request of Dr. James Andrews, the orthopedic surgeon whom I introduced to Hank in 1979 and became the consultant for the Braves. Hank did not like to fly on small planes, so Dr. Andrews asked me to rent a nice car to drive Hank the

Greg Johnson

more than two hours to Birmingham. We were able to talk about our almost twenty years of experience together on the way over and back from the meeting. I was grateful to Hank for giving me the chance to work in baseball, and it was a wonderful opportunity to talk about those years with him one last time.

My work in Greenwood and Savannah got me noticed, and my life got pretty confusing and chaotic. I would work at Savannah most of the season, then get called up to Atlanta for the some of spring training. It's the kind of story that not every sports fan gets to hear, but it's part of the career of anyone who chooses to spend their life playing ballgames.

FOUR

PINCH-HITTING

I t was in 1980 that I got my first opportunity to go to major league spring training. I'm a Florida guy, so it was great to be back in West Palm Beach, but it was better to work with Bobby Cox, my manager, who was the one of the all-time greats. He knew everybody's name and treated everybody fabulous—from the ball boys to the trainers to the big name guys. Cox is one of my favorite baseball people ever.

I was lucky to watch the development of sports medicine, though I wish we knew then what we know now about how to stay healthy. Let's talk about weight training again. Like I said earlier, when I first started playing sports and then working as a trainer, weight training was never encouraged. In fact, we were told not to lift weights. The coaches didn't want players to become so bulky and inflexible that they couldn't perform well on the field. Though the 1960s and especially in the 1970s, that thinking changed, and coaches started to require that athletes do weight training to get stronger so they could actually perform better. We also learned that a stronger athlete could recover faster. Mostly, we would have athletes lift weights along with some basic calisthenics, but it's easy to develop bad habits when lifting, and it's especially easy to get sloppy in your lifting technique when you're getting tired, and that's when you can hurt yourself. That's why a lot of trainers were excited by one of the new ways to get stronger, a machine called the Nautilus, which isolated muscle groups so the training could be safer and more focused.

The Braves were paying attention to the new machines, and by 1980 I was the first to set up the Nautilus program for them. Even then, a lot of the coaches said, "Oh, no, you don't want to lift weights. It's going to ruin your mechanics." But now I had this all set up, and I was in there to help the players work out on the machines. The first guy who walked in was Gaylord Perry, future Hall of Fame pitcher. Perry was known for throwing a spitball, usually with some sort of oily, greasy substance (there are stories told about both Vaseline and K-Y Jelly). He would hide it in different places, like the brim of his cap or on his belt. He mostly got away with it, but he got a lot of batters mad in the process. The Nautilus room was empty when he walked in, so I was excited to see someone—and especially excited to see him. He came in, looked around, and said, "Can I use the machines now?"

"Mr. Perry," I said, "the machines are all greased up and ready to go."

"'All greased up'?" he said. "You had to say 'all greased up'?"

I was so nervous, I thought I was going to pee my pants. I managed to say, "I'm sorry, Mr. Perry."

"Don't worry, kid. I was just messing with you," he said. "Everybody knew I used it."

And then he did his work-out. When he was done, he picked up his gear, and, as he walked out, he winked at me like he was just busting my chops. That was my first experience with a major leaguer on the Nautilus machines.

That first spring training was pretty great, but something better was waiting at the end of the season. After the minor league season was over, I got the call to help out with the big-league team. That call happens to a lot of guys, and we had a name for it—a cup of coffee. The rest of the meal is over but you want to hang out a little longer—and you have to drive home—so you get that cup of coffee. It doesn't last long, and you hope it's good, but you're always glad to have it.

So in the fall of 1981, I got called up for my first cup of coffee.

That September and October the Braves were terrible. We were playing at the old Fulton County stadium, and we hardly had any fans in the stands—a couple of grand a night if we were lucky. It was also a pretty rough neighborhood—you could hear gunshots during some games—so that didn't help with attendance.

But none of that mattered to me. I kept thinking, 'I'm here! I'm in the big leagues!'

Like I said, it was just a cup of coffee. When the first pitch of the next season was thrown, I was back in Savannah again.

I even had a shot at being a trainer with the club in 1982. I hadn't been with them very long, but I still got a call from the head office that they wanted to interview me for the big league job after the season. I thought the interview went well, and I knew that I had been doing good work, but I didn't get the job. At the time, I didn't know today why, but a lot of these jobs have politics that go with them, and I remembered a moment from early on that might have played a part in keeping me in South Carolina.

This incident happened during one of my early times helping out with the big league club at the end of the season [this timeline is a little blurry—the story that follows happens before 82, but the story so far says that 82 was the first time working post-season for Atlanta]. We were playing the St. Louis Cardinals in St. Louis, and Phil Niekro came in early because he was the starting pitcher that night. I was there but the head trainer wasn't. Knucksie, which was what everyone called Niekro, said, "Hey, guys, I need a shoulder rubdown."

"Sorry," I told him, "the head trainer's not here. He should be back pretty soon."

Knucksie was heading for the table and said, "I don't care. I'm here. I need a rubdown, and you're going to do it."

Well, what are you going to do? When the team captain tells you he wants a rubdown and wants you to do it, you just do it.

The head trainer showed up about an hour later, after the rubdown was finished.

"Thanks, guys," Knucksie said as we packed up his stuff to head out.

The trainer gave him a look, and Knucksie added, "I got Greg to do the rubdown. And you better watch out, he did a better job than you." And then he walked out the door.

Well, the head trainer gave me a look that shoulda killed me. And that look came back to my mind when I got the message that I didn't get the assistant trainer job with the Atlanta club.

So that job didn't end up happening, yet I still had a great time working in the Bigs even if my yearly schedule—back and forth between Georgia and South Carolina—were complicated. I had a lot of hope, and I was still chasing my dream. I think that the hopes and dreams kept me longer in baseball than I should have stayed. I had promised myself that I'd only stay a few years unless I made it, but I kept going back. Eventually, I would know that I had to make a change. Before we get to that story, though, I want to share some stories about what big league life is like. And I'll start with one of the most important people I worked with.

What can I say about Bobby Cox, except that he was one of the nicest guys I ever met in baseball. He was well liked by all his players, coaches, and staff. He treated everyone with respect and made everyone feel like part of the team.

My first thoughts of Bobby that come to mind was in the summer of 1981 I was up with the "big club" after the minor league season was over. Bobby and I were walking to the dugout through the tunnel in old Fulton County Stadium, and he turned to me and said, "I hope the both of us get to walk this walk a couple of thousand times again in our career."

I stood beside him, taking it all in, and said, "Me too." Though it didn't quite happen that way for me, it sure did for him.

I remember as a kid admiring any Yankee player, and one of them was Bobby, who played second base for the Yankees in the 60s. Bobby told me story after story of playing with Joe Pepitone, Mickey Mantle, Yogi Berra, Bobby Richardson, and Tom Tresh as well as many others. I listened for hours to his stories and thought about how lucky I was to hear these stories directly from a guy who played for the Yankees.

The strange thing about coffee, though, is that the wait staff will keep bringing them to you. The early 80s were like that for me when it came to the bigs because I got called up again in 1982 [we need to get this timeline straightened out—the ATL stats are correct, but the job history is a not as focused].

That year was better. We won the National League West, which was great, but then we got swept by the Cardinals in the National League Championship Series. I had another great couple of weeks with the team, but I wasn't quite so star-struck this time, and I started to form some opinions about the players and coaches that have stayed with me until today.

The Braves' manager at the time was Joe Torre, who was the biggest jerk I'd ever met in my life. He was not very personable, and he also didn't seem to care that much about the team. I remember one game when we were playing in the Astrodome, and we're in a tight game. We had a three-game series with the Astros, and all of them were close. Torre was in the dugout standing next to Bob Gibson, our pitching coach and one of the greatest of all time. I was standing right next to Gibson, and I was hoping for some insights into the game or maybe some great baseball history. Instead, they're checking out some blonde woman in the first row instead of paying attention to the baseball game. And I'm thinking, 'Really?' We lost all three games. That was the first of his three seasons with the Braves, and the best they had with him as the skipper.

Like Torre, Bob Gibson—we all called him Gibby—was not a very personable individual. He wouldn't do autographs, really didn't like the press, and was pretty aloof. I remember him not understanding how pitching didn't come as naturally to the Braves pitchers as it did for him. He was many of the superstars that never really made a good coach. Hank Aaron once told me that Gibby was one of two pitchers that he feared as a hitter because, as Hank said, "Gibby would just as soon hit you as throw a strike."

On my first road trip to St. Louis to play the Cardinals, the team made Tommie Aaron and me roommates. I had first met Tommie in spring training a few years earlier, and we got along great. Tommie was very different from his brother Hank. He was more outgoing and had a great sense of humor. I guess you'd have to be if your older brother was Hank Aaron. But between the two of them, they hit more home runs than any other brother team in history. On the trip, Tommie and I talked about how much fun it was to be to be on the first winning team in Atlanta Braves history.

Tommie was one of the nicest men I ever met in baseball, very approachable and an overall great person. But he died just a few years later, in 1984, of leukemia. The baseball world lost a great ambassador that day.

We called Hall of Famer Phil Niekro "pops" or "grand-dad" because he was in his forties. Sports always has a lot of young guys! He was in his early forties at the time and played until he was forty-eight. Knucksie was the second-best pitcher I saw in my baseball career. He was a knuckleball pitcher—which explains the nickname—and could have won more than 318 games if he had played on better teams. In twenty-four seasons, he only went to the playoffs twice.

Knucksie was a team captain, which was an official position, and the judge in the kangaroo court that we had with the Braves, which was not an official position. What did the court do? For example, you could get fined for "stupid" plays, and Knucksie decided who was guilty and what they had to pay.

I don't know if it was because Knucksie was old enough not to give a damn or if throwing a crazy pitch for his whole career, but something made him a leader for team shenanigans. One day in Montreal we had a team party and all the rookie players, including myself, had to dress up as women. We had on wigs, dresses, panty hose, makeup, the whole works. The team then sent us out of the hotel to get something to prove we actually went out in public. The guys paired me with Ken Dayley, a rookie pitcher, and we were told to go out and buy a book at the bookstore across the street from the hotel. I've had more fun at a dentist's office. After getting the book and returning to the party, we had to serve the players their food and drinks. The big fun for them was that they made us drink what we mixed if they didn't like what we made. None of the players liked the drink I made, and I don't think any of us rookies made a single drink that they did like. Phil was the one directing the whole night. It was great fun and a lot of laughs, even if the next day was pretty terrible.

Phil Niekro was a great guy, and a veteran we learned a lot from, but we had others around the Braves, too. In 1982 Chris Chambliss was the Braves first basemen, and, in my opinion, he was a huge part of our success in our drive to championship baseball. As a bonus, it was a pleasure to be a teammate with a true Yankee legend.

Chris had playoff and World Series experience with the Yankees, while we had little or no post-season experience with our young team. Chris brought this knowledge to the club. He was a class act and talked of his experiences as a winner in major league baseball. He taught the young guys a lot about winning, though the post season didn't last long for us that year. Chris was very humble and liked helping the young players.

I remember flying from Atlanta to our west coast trip in 1982. My seat on the charter was next to Chris, and we spoke for hours about Yankee history. I told him that Mickey Mantle was my hero growing up and that the first baseball game I ever saw was the Yankees playing in Washington against the Senators. He thrilled me with stories of his experiences with such Yankee greats as Mickey, Bobby Richardson, Frankie Crosetti, Yogi Berra, Joe DiMaggio, and many more.

One night in Houston, Tommy Boggs was on the mound pitching against Nolan Ryan. In the top of the first inning, after striking out our first two batters and Dale Murphy then struck out on three pitches, Dale came back to the dugout and said, "Boys it's going to be a long night," and sure enough it was. We lost, and Ryan struck out something like fifteen batters while going the entire nine innings.

Ryan was the greatest pitcher I personally watched play baseball during my career. He was famous for his 100 MPH fastball, but the hitters who faced him will tell you he had a great curve ball that was just as much an out pitch as his heater.

Baseball is great entertainment, but sometimes you need a little something extra to put asses in the seats. The minor leagues had Max Patkin and other guys like him, but the Bigs also had their non-player star attractions. And in San Diego, that was Ted Giannoulas, the San Diego Chicken, probably the greatest entertainment sidekick in baseball history. He was great at making kids laugh, and he was great at making umpires upset. He was making huge appearance dollars when I saw him perform in the minor leagues as well as the Bigs. Outside the uniform Ted was a good guy and a pleasure to be around.

But you could find good guys wearing a uniform, too. One of the three best human beings I've ever met in my life—in addition to Archie Griffin and Bobby Bowden—was Dale Murphy. Dale was a devout Mormon when most religious players seemed to put their religion ahead of their game. Murph was one guy who was able to find the right balance, and he was one of the hardest working players I every witnessed. He was a two-time National League Player of the Year and our team captain. You might expect a devoutly religious guy to get the cold shoulder, but Murph was loved by his teammates. I never heard a bad word about him. Players respected him so much that no one ever used a curse word within shouting distance of Murph. Even when I was in the minors, Murph always talked with me and treated me like teammate.

The best story I heard about Murph was one year he went into Ted Turner's office and offered to give back some of his salary from the year before because he thought he had a bad year. Ted said no. If they had a Hall of Fame for great people who played baseball, Dale Murphy would be in on a landslide ballot his first year.

I always remembered how good Murph was to every-body—big league or not. I tried to follow his example and treat everyone fairly and help them get in better condition or rehab safely. Sure, it was a great feeling to be able to help guys like Phil Niekro or Steve Bedrosian get healthy and stay strong, but I always wanted all the guys to get better and keep playing.

Baseball lets you meet a lot of people. Some are great people, and some are great friends. Brett Butler was a good friend, and we both were in the Show for the first time in the early 80s. Butler had made it on the Braves in 1981, but they still hadn't figured out what to do with him the next year, and he would be traded the year after that.

I remember sitting in the dugout with him when Brett said, "I have as much of a chance playing tonight as you do, Greg." He was pretty frustrated at that point, but he went on to have a great career.

Another fun detail from that era of the Braves was that we had a pretty amazing-looking charter plane. Air Nigeria had ordered a bunch of planes and painted them to match their flag. But either the airline never made it or they decided not to buy this one plane, so the Braves got a sweet deal on leasing that plane during the playoffs. Somehow, Brett and I were always on that charter plane together.

While you expect to meet a lot of athletes and owners in sports, you don't necessarily expect to meet other celebrities. But famous people are a lot like everyone else, and they like sports. Someone I never expected to come in contact with was Olivia Newton-John.

Newton-John was on a world tour, still supporting her big album, Physical. She came to watch us play and was brought into the locker-room before the game. I don't know why she came to see the game—she's from Australia, and I didn't think baseball was huge in Australia. She showed up wearing tight, black-leather pants, and she was both sexy and nice. She spoke to everyone that came up to her, which was everyone. She was one of the most famous people in movies and music at the time, and we all wanted to meet her.

One of our pitchers, Steve Bedrosian, went up to her and said, "Hey, babe, want to hook up after the game?"

She looked at him and said, "Honey, you couldn't handle this!" That got a lot of laughs.

When she left, one of her tour manager brought us a box full of long-sleeve, tour t-shirts. I kept mine for years.

Even with all the distractions, we won the West title on the last day of the season in San Diego. We lost to the Padres

1-5 that game, but the Giants beat the Dodgers in LA on a Joe Morgan late-inning home run. We had a wild party in the locker room after the game. The Braves hadn't won the pennant since 1969, and we knew what it would mean to our fans, but it meant even more to the players. And that party included plenty of beer and Champagne, though the Champagne has a great story to go with it. I'm not sure that even the players know this one.

Ted Turner bought cases of Dom Perignon Champagne to celebrate. Apparently he didn't know how much it cost; he just liked the stuff. When he found out it was about $100 per bottle at the time, he made the traveling secretary, Bill Acree, go out and buy the cheap stuff for the celebration in the locker room so he could save the good stuff for himself and the managers. I stole a bottle and kept it for over twenty years before I finally drank it.

After the game we flew to St. Louis and got rained out. First game Phil Niekro pitched and we had the Cardinals beat 1-0 into the top of the 5th inning; then the rain started, and we couldn't finish the game.

We ended up getting swept by the Cards. They went on to beat the Milwaukee Brewers in the World Series.

It was a first for Atlanta though, the first championship for the city in any sport. It was my second biggest thrill in my professional baseball career to stand on that white line and be introduced to over 50,000 fans and a TV audience of millions. Of course, my biggest thrill in baseball was meeting Mickey Mantle. But I know that a lot fewer people get to have the experience of lining up for playoff game in the Bigs.

Working with the big league club was great, but I still had a couple more years to go with the Braves organization. The Savannah team moved upstate to Greenville, SC, at the end of the 1983 season, and I moved with them. I still had two more seasons in baseball, but I could see that I was either going to have to keep fighting to move up or look somewhere else for a better opportunity.

I had seen how weight and resistance training was helping skilled athletes, and I kept wanting to learn more about how to help players get better and stay healthy. My years in Greenville would help with that, and I still had a chance to spend time with the game I loved.

FIVE

CHANGEUP:
BASEBALL, FOOTBALL, AND
THE LONG BALL

At the end of the day, sports is just a business. You see people's lives turned upside down because they get released, or they don't get a contract, or they get hurt and they can't play anymore. It's tough because you see them every day, and then you don't. And it's like getting a divorce every season. People come into your life, become your teammate, drinking buddy, friend, and then they leave at the end of the season. Or even partway through. It's hard, though. It's probably the hardest part. It's kind of like life, everybody goes their separate ways, and sometimes you stay in relationships—you stay friends, you catch up over beers after games—and sometimes you don't. They just become another face in the crowd.

The beginning of 1985 was the beginning of the end for me in baseball. It was my turn to be the guy who goes away. It wasn't an easy year or an easy process, but I still had some good times during that last season. And I found a great, new path forward.

First, though, I want to talk about one of my scariest moments. It was at the end of the '85 season during winter ball, and it involves Bob Veale, Hank Aaron, and a rising star, Ron Gant.

Bob Veale was one of the most intimidating pitchers in National League history. Bob was funny, strong, and really understood minor league players. He was also one of the kindest individuals I ever met in professional baseball. He would throw batting practice for hours and was a baseball man through and through. Bob was the only other pitcher that Hank Aaron said he feared besides Bob Gibson, because, like Gibson, Bob was not afraid to throw at a batter. He was also huge, and his size and fearlessness came in handy with some of the young guys on the team.

Veale's strength was especially useful when Ron Gant got into trouble.

Ronnie was a guy who loved to go out and have fun even though the players had a curfew. One night, Gant was out dancing after hours, and at some point a woman came on to him and wanted to dance. Ron, being more than happy to entertain an attractive woman, started dancing with her. She never told him about a boyfriend. So the boyfriend showed up drunk and got all pissed off and wanted to fight. Of course, the last guy you want to fight is Ron Gant. He's built like a brick shithouse.

But the boyfriend wouldn't back off, so they started to mix it up out in the parking lot. Ronnie proceeded to beat the shit out of him. As I understand it, the boyfriend's buddy went to his car, got a gun, came back, and fired it into the ground. The bullet ricocheted and hit Ronnie in the leg. He started to bleed pretty bad because the bullet hit near his artery. The buddy then shot again before the fight got broken up.

That was when I got a call looking for Eddie Haas, who was in charge. At least, he was supposed to be in charge, but he was out somewhere. He didn't last long after that night.

I answered the phone because Eddie and I were rooming together. I said, "Who is this?"

A man on the other end of the line said, "This is St. Francis Hospital. We believe we've got a couple of your ballplayers here, though one didn't give his real name."

"How bad is it?"

"One of them is getting his last rights read to him," he said.

The guy lived, and so did Ronnie.

I had to call Hank Aaron the next day. I never saw him that mad—before or after. Hank didn't show a lot of emotion, but my God was he mad. He got down there, and he brought Bob Veale with him. Bob was 6'6", 250 pounds, and he grabbed Gant, picked him up, and pinned him up against the wall. He held Gant there while Hanks read him the riot act.

Aaron said, "Give me one good reason I don't release your sorry ass right now."

Gant was scared as hell. He said, "If you tell Bob to put me down, I'll tell you."

Bob let go of him.

And then Gant said, "Because I'm going to be one of the best damn players you've ever had in your life."

Hank took a minute to look at him and said, "You better be."

Gant went home to Texas after that to heal up, and he struggled early on before becoming a great player.

It was around then that I was asked to go to the airport to pick up the Braves' new baseball manager, Chuck Tanner. During our short time together that winter, Chuck asked about my position, the team, the players, and overall thoughts on the Atlanta Braves as an organization. He was personable, talkative, and engaging. I would have loved to have worked with Chuck for a while, but my days were coming to an end with the Braves.

Another great person I got to meet that winter was Tom Glavine. At the time I met him, Glavine was a promising left-handed, 19-year-old pitcher. From the first time I saw him pitch, I thought he was going to be a good one. We were

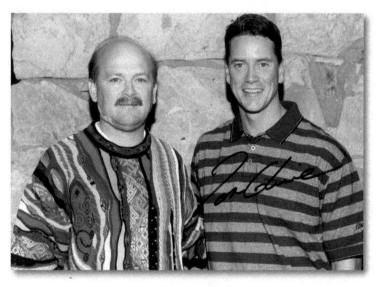

Greg with Tom Glavin

teammates only for that short winter ball year, but Tommie and I played a lot of golf together after I left the Braves.

Glavine is always in the conversation of best pitchers ever. Another guy who had great stuff was Bert Blyleven, who pitched for both the Minnesota Twins and the Cleveland Indians.

But the best pitcher I ever saw—and I still say that to this day—was Nolan Ryan.

Nolan Ryan would just scare guys. I always go back to that game in Houston when Boggs was pitching for us. Boggs was a decent pitcher, and he was doing ok. Then Ryan got to the mound and threw heat up around 101 or 102. Maybe he threw harder, but the JUGS guns weren't around too much back then. That was the night that Dale Murphy, came back to the dugout, and said, "Boys, it's going to be a long night." Murphy had one hit, one walk, scored one run and went on to win the MVP award that year, so you had to listen to him.

We lost a close one. Boggs had a solid game. But Ryan was in another category. When he had his stuff—or even close to it—he was unhittable. He should have a better won/loss record, and the only reason he doesn't is because he played for lousy teams—the California Angels, the Houston Astros, and the Texas Rangers. He won the World Series with the Mets, but that was early on. Imagine what he could have done with a solid defense behind him and great hitting at the plate.

After all my years with the Braves organization, I could see that I was never going to move up. Maybe it was political, maybe it was something else, but the time had come for me to find another place to work. It's never an easy thing, leaving a job. And I had a great time with the Braves—the minor league teams as well as the major league club—which made the decision even harder. I had learned a lot, though, because I had good mentors and had listened to them, so I knew that I could go a lot of different places with my skills as a trainer. I had also made a lot of good connections, which were important as I started to plan out my next move. Once again, my home state proved to be a key part of my network.

Through my connections at Florida State, I was asked to help with the United States Football League (USFL) Jacksonville Bulls during two-a-days and preseason in 1985. My old roommate, Randy Oravetz, had gotten a call from one of his former athletic trainers who was the head trainer for the Bulls, and Randy told that guy to reach out to me. Of course, I accepted, and I began a new life as an athletic trainer in professional football.

The USFL was a short-lived venture that was supposed to compete with the NFL. The idea was for them to be a spring/summer league so that fans could still watch football when college and professional ball wasn't being played. The league lasted three seasons, and I was involved for just a short time right before the last season they played. Turns out that competing with the NFL isn't a great idea.

The head coach for Jacksonville was Lindy Infante, and the general manager was Larry Csonka, the great Miami Dolphins fullback. And let me tell you, they were tough guys. Those three months were the hardest of my professional career. The days were from dawn to oh-dark-thirty every day of the week.

Because it was a spring and summer league, the offseason was during the winter, and that winter ended up being one of the coldest in Jacksonville history. We had a few days during practice when it never got above freezing.

But I had a chance to meet some great football players. Some of the guys that still stand out to me are Brian Sipe (NFL Player of the Year with the Cleveland Browns in 1980), Archie Griffin (the only two-time winner of the Heisman Trophy, 1974 and 1975), and Mike Rozier (Heisman Trophy winner, 1983).

Brian Sipe was our quarterback and a true gentleman. He dressed like a fashion model, and you would have guessed he was a lawyer or a businessman instead of a professional football player. He led by example, not by words. He treated me very well, and I will always remember him as a man of great class. The players were always being rushed around to different meetings or off for drills, but Brian always had time to say hello and thank everyone in the organization—not just his teammates and coaches. And I remember that the wait staff at the local restaurants were always happy to see him because he left great tips and treated them with respect, which isn't always the case with famous football players.

As much as Brian was a great guy, Archie Griffin was one of the three best human beings I've ever met—in or out of sports. He treated everyone around him with respect, and it did matter if it was another player, a clubhouse guy, or a lowly trainer like me. Archie always had time to talk during camp, and he would ask what I needed, which was a big change from most other players, and when we went out for dinner or drinks he always picked up the tab. We had some great conversations! He played for seven seasons with the Bengals before he was with the Bulls, and everyone looked up to him for being an NFL veteran. And he tried to be a mentor to Mike Rozier, another Heisman winner.

I always love to ask this trivia question: what was the only backfield in the history of professional football that three Heisman Trophys? Nobody ever names the Jacksonville Bulls of the USFL, but Archie Griffin had two and Mike Rozier had one. Which meant that even though the Bulls had two running backs, they had three Heismans between them. That's an answer that usually has sports fans reaching for their phones!

Of course, when you start to talk about running backs, you have to talk about Larry Csonka. I remember being impressed by his nose. It had been broken so many times, it was just this grotesque presence in the middle of this face. Zonk was the toughest football player I ever saw, one of the toughest ever, but I think Jacksonville recruited him because of his name and not GM skills. He was a fair guy, just not very personable.

I remember that Coach Lindy Infante was really a taskmaster. He was the head coach and ended up becoming the head coach for the Green Bay Packers after the USFL folded. I learned one of my biggest lessons from Coach, and it had to do with going to meetings. We had a lot of team meeting, and everybody went to the team meetings the medical staff gave to get updates on the players. You know, the "who's got this injury and who's got that" kind of meeting. I was supposed to be there because I'm part of the team doing the medical updates. So I walked in probably less than a minute late. Everybody else was in there and I said to myself, "Oh shit."

I looked around and Coach Infante said, "Greg, come here."

I walked down, and he said, "You're late to my meeting."

"I'm sorry."

He said, "You're either horseshit, or you don't give a damn. Which is it?"

The next fifteen seconds were probably the longest fifteen seconds of my life. Sixty people or more were watching me, and I just kept thinking, "Oh shit, oh shit, oh shit." But I finally pulled myself together and said, "Well, Coach, I guess I'm just horseshit today." Because I didn't want to say I didn't give a damn.

Infante gave me a long look and said, "Go sit down." And I did.

So my life lesson was this: don't be late. To this day, I'm not late to meetings. In fact, I'm there early most of the time. For me, it's about respect. That's the lesson I learned, to be respectful of other people's time: to show that you give a shit, show up on time.

I learned a lot from the team sports I was part of for fifteen years. I learned to understand my teammates, and to do that I had to develop my empathy for them. A lot of guys came from very different backgrounds from mine, and I had to sort of get out of my own way to really hear what their lives were like. These were almost always young guys who were struggling to make it, and I really respected their drive and dedication. And I learned to like a lot of things I didn't ever expect to like—like country music and rap.

It's easy to think that you're some hot shit if you're part of a ball club, but I learned that the guys who really succeeded were humble. Or mostly so. They listened to coaches and teammates about how to get better, stronger. And we all had to rely on each other to improve throughout a season and a career. Even the greats had to put in the hours and the work. You have to pay your dues to succeed, and all of us who had any kind of success in sports paid their dues.

We're always connected to something that's bigger than us. I loved being part of the history of baseball, learning the stories, meeting the legends of the game. But when the time came, I knew I had to move on and start a new chapter. As someone who loved the game of golf, I couldn't have been happier with what happened next. Even if I still had some more dues to pay.

SIX

GOING GREEN:
LIFE ON THE PGA TOUR 1985-87

To tell you what happened next, I need to go back a year.

I was back in Greenville through the end of the 1984 season, and I knew that I needed to make a change. I had stalled out, but I didn't know what to do next. It was after the season, and I was hanging around in Greenville when I got a call from a guy I had known from the Braves but hadn't seen in a while, Glenn Diamond. He had just gotten the job as the executive producer of PGA Tour Entertainment, and he was calling to give me a heads up. He knew that I was a big golfer and had loved the game since I started playing in high school. He wanted to let me know that the PGA Tour was putting together a fitness truck to follow the players to the Tour spots. Just in case I was interested.

I said, "Hell, yes, I'm interested. Are you kidding?"

"No, it's for real," he said, "And I can get you the name and number of the guy you need to talk to. Just let me know."

As I was writing down some notes about the job, Glenn told me that they had already hired one other person, Gene Lane. Lane has also been a minor league trainer with the Braves and a friend of mine.

I want to give some context for what was happening. It was the mid-80s, and athletic training remained in early development. Sure, the baseball and football guys had really started to come around, but golf was still considered such a finesse sport that any conditioning exercises or weight-training regimen were actively avoided. Golfers were told that any of that stuff was going to ruin their swing. This fitness truck the Tour was putting together was revolutionary, and it took a while to really gather steam. It wasn't until Tiger Woods got serious about bulking up that weight training became part of mainstream golf.

But I had seen what conditioning and weight training could do for other finesse athletes like pitchers. Offering this kind of support to golfers was pretty exciting, and I was stoked to think that I could be part of something new.

Right after I put down the phone with Diamond, I called Lane to see if he wouldn't mind if we teamed up on the fitness truck.

He immediately said, "Hey, yeah. That'd be great!"

I called Glenn back, and he gave me the name and number I needed to call to contact the fitness truck sponsor. The sponsor was DP Fitness, famous for their inexpensive exercise equipment. The name Glenn gave me was for Lanier Johnson, which, with the last name "Johnson," I took as a good omen.

I immediately called this other Johnson, and he asked if I could be at Ponte Vedra Beach, Florida that Monday.

Absolutely.

That Monday, right on time, I walked into the office of Lanier Johnson. The guy was as bald as a cue ball. We had a great conversation, and, at the end of the day, they offered me the job.

As soon as I got back to Greenville, I told the Braves that I was done. I had been with the organization since 1978, and that was enough. I was disappointed to step away from baseball, but I know I wasn't the only guy in history who struggled with that decision. The disappointment was easier to swallow for me, though, because I was going on to work in another sport I loved. This work ended up being the greatest job I've ever had—bar none. I got to work with Jack Nicklaus, Arnold Palmer, and Tom Watson, as well as Payne Stewart, who ended up being one of my best friends. Such good friends, in fact, that I named my daughter Chelsea after his.

I started off talking about how much I loved baseball but I never got big enough to play it competitively. I did find a sport that I could play, though, and that was golf. So I had played high school golf but really got into it in college. At Florida State I met Jeff Sluman, Kenny Knox, and Paul Azinger who were all on the golf team. They were pretty good, and they really helped me keep my skills sharp. And they're still friends of mine today.

If I could have had one career that I didn't have, it would have been to be a professional golfer. I loved golf. I still do today. It's the greatest sport in the world because it's the only sport in the world that does one thing: If you don't play well, you don't get paid. If you don't make the cut, you get zero. And here's the bad news, you have to pay an entry fee. It doesn't matter if you're Jack Nicklaus or Tiger Woods, you have to pay an entry fee. You have to pay your own expenses. You have to pay your lodging, your food, your caddy, your travel. So you have to put out all this money upfront, which can be quite a bit, and if you don't make the cut, you don't get paid. I love that team sports means that you have—literally—a team around you. It's a good feeling to have teammates and work together. But I love that feeling of being out on the course and it's just you and the land, your skills and that goddamned ball. While you learn a lot about the world on a team, you learn a lot about yourself on a golf course.

So now I was done with the Braves, done with the USFL, and joining the PGA Tour. Not the Tour itself, of course, but I was part of the game.

Then reality hit.

The guy who hired me said, "You're going to have to drive a tractor trailer."

Now, I had driven some big vehicles. As part of the minor league organization, I had driven a lot of different things, including the bus we used for away games. But nothing as large as a big rig. I wasn't looking forward to it, but I figured I could learn how to handle a semi.

Then he said something that was a great relief, "You won't have to drive it on long trips. We'll hire a contract driver for that."

The truck ended up being a forty-two-foot tractor-trailer. Three of us were going to get the training: Paul Callaway, Gene Lane, and me. We all packed up our stuff, and they flew us to Jacksonville in late 1985.

Our training took place at an abandoned air force base outside of Jacksonville. We drove up to the office they had set up at this truck driver training school, got out, and stood around, not quite sure what to do. Pretty soon three dudes walked up, all of them chewing tobacco, wearing cowboy boots and the raunchiest clothing you've ever seen. I looked over at Paul Callaway, who's from LA, and he was wearing Gucci shoes, a pair of dress slacks, and a five-hundred-dollar cashmere sweater.

The roughest looking one walked over, looked at Paul, and said, "Boy, that shit ain't working here."

Luckily I had on a pair of jeans, tennis shoes, a t-shirt, and a jeans jacket. So they barely looked at me before we started walking out to where the trucks were parked.

One of the guys stopped me and pointed, "This is your truck, boy. Get in."

You want to talk about some dues to pay? For the next two weeks, for eight hours a day, we drove around on that abandoned air force base. All during that time I was thinking, "What the hell did I get myself into?" I had driven pickups and buses, and I knew how to drive a stick, but not something with eighteen gears. It wasn't like there were just ten different positions, either. There were switches and toggles and different clutch positions, too. It was a lot of stuff to think about, and a lot of patterns to keep track of and memorize.

At the end of each day, though, I thought, "This is what I want. And if I want to do this, then these are the dues I have to pay. And I'm going to do it." I'd been working with dedicated, driven athletes for a long time, and I knew that sometimes you just had to do drills so you could get where you wanted to be.

After that two weeks, we went to pick up the trailers that were going to be accompanying the Tour. They were getting their final updates in Atlanta, and we needed to drive them to Palm Springs, CA, for the start of the 1986 season. True to their word, they hired a contract driver for the long haul, but I wanted to ride along to see what it was all about. When I got out of that truck cab to Palm Springs three days later, I was so worn out that I slept for two days. I don't know how that guy did it. He drank a lot of coffee, but I have a feeling that wasn't the only thing he was taking to stay awake. He let me take a couple of short shifts, but mostly I just watched the road or slept in the back where we had a sleeper and a refrigerator.

When I finally woke up, I walked out into the bright sun and a new career in golf.

The big rig dues were worth it almost immediately. My first event was the Bob Hope Desert Classic. The second night we were there, they had an event at Bob Hope's house. I was still pretty young, and I didn't expect to be included in any of the special events, so I was blown away when I found out that I was invited to the evening at the Hope's home. And even though I had been around big name sports figures, it was still an awesome thrill to meet Bob and Delores Hope. Bob's wife greeted everyone upon showing up that night and was truly a very kind woman. Bob couldn't have been nicer. He had clearly heard about the exercise trailer, and, when we met, he said, "Man, I want to come in and see that van." I told him he should drop by, but I thought he'd be busy with the tournament, and we'd never see him.

I was wrong. True to his word, he came in during the tournament to have a look around. Over the years, we would have a lot of celebrities—as well as the golfers—come to visit the truck. In the early days, we didn't know whether anybody was going to come in or not, so we were pretty glad to have our first visitor.

The first guy who walked in was Tom Kite. He said that he just wanted to see the truck.

He looked around and asked, "Do you have a bike?"

"Yeah," I said, "We have a bike."

He nodded. "Great. I'll come in after my round."

It was funny—of course we had a bike! We had all the fitness equipment, and we had all the rehab equipment. In the early days, we had all the stuff in just one trailer. We even had a state-of-the-art Sony TV in that thing. The DP Fitness guys told us the TV was the first flat screen ever made. Or maybe it was the first flat screen available outside Sony. Either way, it was a pretty awesome piece of equipment. It might have been our most popular piece of equipment for a while, to be honest.

We had a hell of a time setting the place up, though. We had set up a special air conditioning unit, get all the equipment ready, and wire up the Sony. It took us the whole week to get it ready, but it was a hit. We had twenty players a day in there, and everybody loved it. We got better doing the set up as the season went on, and the players really came to rely on the trailer as a place to escape the heat and the fans. Don't get me wrong, the fans are important, but the players always liked a bit of privacy during the tournaments.

In addition to learning how to drive the semi and set up the equipment, I had to learn a different part of the training and rehab trade. In baseball, it was all bad elbows, bad shoulders, and bad knees. In golf it was bad necks and bad backs. I'd say that about seventy-five percent of the injuries I dealt with were bad backs. It's because of the repetition, not because of poor swing mechanics like you get with amateur golfers. With professional golfers, it's repetition. Sooner or later on the golf tour, everybody who is out there long enough to even get a cup of coffee will have a back problem.

I had to go somewhere and learn more about how to treat backs. I mean, backs are a bit more complicated than knees and elbows. Since I had time off after the USFL training camp, I thought it would be a good time to add to my skillset. So I went to the San Francisco Spine Institute, which was one of the foremost clinics in the country. I spent some time up there in the fall of 1985 learning how to treat spine issues before I started working with the Tour.

Another complication was age. In baseball (and briefly football), it was all these fairly young guys, but golf lets you play until you're a lot older. So I was treating guys from the age of twenty on up to Sam Snead, who was 65 when I was working with him. I had to learn a different way to do things.

When we had the trailer all set up, we were equipped to take care of backs. I became great at manual manipulation. We called manual therapy the million-dollar roll. You put them on their side and roll them over. And they hear all that popping and they love it. Then I would say something like, "Now, let's do something to strengthen that back."

The audible popping isn't much, really. It's just a shifting of gas—like popping your knuckles. In most instances, it's really not doing a whole lot. Sometimes you get things inside that need to pop back into place, but it's mostly for show. The athletes, though, they hear it, and they get this endorphin release, and they think it's doing something. Then they'll listen to you when you tell them how to keep their backs strong.

The most important person in the fitness trailer was Dr. Frank Jobe. He was the medical director for the trailer during my days with the PGA Tour, and it was an honor to work with the man who developed the Tommy John procedure. I had met Dr. Jobe while I was a trainer with the Braves, but I got to know him better during the Tour. At first I was a little amused that he would come into the trailer and fall asleep a lot, but then I found out he was taking medicine for a sleeping disorder he had. He was a good man and always treated me with respect and kindness.

The great thing about the fitness trailer was that we got close to all these great golfers, but we were also just kind of behind the scenes. We were the guys who helped the players get out and do their thing. We were invisible to the fans, but we were right there at the center of the events, and the players relied on us.

Greg Johnson

I remember the 1986 Masters, when Jack Nicklaus won his last golf tournament ever. His comeback at that Masters is probably the greatest golf comeback story this side of Tiger Woods after his back surgeries. Nicklaus came back into the fitness truck after the tournament was over, and he said, "You know, you really helped me. My back's been bad all week, but you've kept me going." And he was in that truck every day, so we knew what was going on. When you're part of something that great, it makes you feel good to know that you were able to help somebody.

So I'd like to share some stories of the guys who came through our fancy trailer. Some of them were real friends, some I only met once or twice, but we had some good times, and I'm proud of the work I did to help a lot of golfers stay on the course.

I spent a lot of time with Payne Stewart in the fitness van during the 1985-90 seasons. The younger golfers as well as the older players—guys like Jack Nicklaus, Arnold Palmer, and Raymond Floyd—admired him. They admired him for his play on the course as well as who he was as a person.

What a lot of people don't necessarily know is that Payne was a very big practical joker. At the Memorial Tournament in 1988 Payne came into the fitness van and said, "Greg, I've got to take a shit."

I said, "Payne, you know there's no bathroom in the van."

After conceding that there was no bathroom in the van, Payne headed into the locker room to put on his workout gear. Curtis Strange was already in the trailer face down on one of the treatment tables getting an e-stim and a heat pack

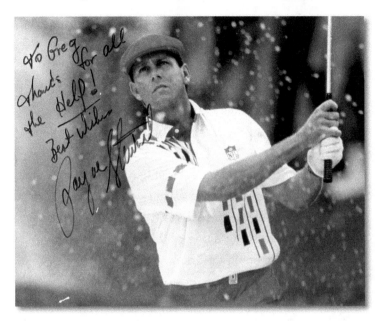

Payne Stewart

on his back. A few minutes later Payne Stewart came out dressed to run on the treadmill.

The next thing I heard was a yell from Strange, "You son of a bitch!"

Curtis jumped up off the table and chased Payne out of the van. Payne laughed the whole way out. Payne had taken a shit in a locker-room trashcan and placed it under the hole in the treatment table where Curtis was lying. While Payne and Strange were still running around outside, back in the van I was laughing so hard that I was on the floor. The next day, Curtis super-glued the shoe trees in Payne's golf shoes as payback.

One day during the US Open in 1988, Payne and I were talking about children's names since I had found out that I was going to be a dad earlier that year.

Payne said, "Gee why don't you name your child Chelsea?" Payne's daughter was named Chelsea. I really liked the idea and suggested it to my wife. We both loved the name, and the rest is history.

Speaking of Curtis Strange, I met him in 1986, and I really didn't think much of him. He wasn't very out-going, and it was six months or so before we really started getting along. I now consider Curtis to be one of the nicest but most misunderstood gentlemen on the Tour.

One of my favorite memories of Curtis happened in 1988 during the US Open. The week had been an awesome experience at Brookline. The last day of the tournament, I was packing up the van getting ready to head to Memphis, and Curtis walked in and said, "Hey, Greg, can I hang out here until its time for me to practice?"

Curtis and I played Mean 18 Golf on the computer to pass the time. He said that he couldn't sleep at the hotel and that all the people in the locker room were a distraction. We had a policy that no press, family, or caddies were allowed in the van. Our van was one of the few places of peace for the players, and they could do and say whatever they wanted.

When it was time for Curtis to practice and get ready for his day—and after I beat him in eighteen holes of golf on the computer (something later that day the second-best player of the week, Nick Faldo, couldn't do on the course)—I felt that just maybe I helped him in a small way to win the greatest golf tournament in the world.

It turns out that Curtis had a reputation for being cheap, and I have the perfect story to illustrate that cheap streak.

After winning the US Open in 1989 for the second time in two years, he was in the fitness truck during the St. Jude Classic Tournament in Memphis. I was congratulating him on the win and asked where he was staying that week.

Strange said, "I'm staying at the Red Roof Inn."

"Curtis, you've got to be shitting me," I said. "The Red Roof Inn? You cheapskate!"

"I'm staying in the suite," he said.

"There are no suites at the Red Roof Inn," I told him. "And I know that because that's where I'm staying, too."

But Strange was also an intense competitor, and I have a great story about that, too. It was the BellSouth Classic Tournament in Atlanta. I was heading into the locker-room for lunch, and I walked by Curtis on his way to the tenth tee. I said, "Hello, Curtis." He said nothing and acted like I wasn't even there.

After the day was over, Curtis came into the van, and I said, "Hey, Curtis, why were you such an ass to me, not saying 'hi' back near the tenth tee?"

He shook his head, "I didn't see you, man."

This story is why I consider him one of the most intense competitors I ever saw. The only other two players that I saw who were even close were Jack Nicklaus and Raymond Floyd.

Curtis and I see each other every once in a while, and talk about "crapper" Payne Stewart and how much we truly miss our friend.

I've mentioned before that one of the amazing things about being in the sports world is meeting your heros. I can't believe how lucky I was to meet Mickey Mantle, but I only had the one evening to talk with him. I'm incredibly lucky to have gotten to know Jack Nicklaus really well. Jack was just a class act. In fact, he taught me another one of the biggest life lesson I've ever learned.

"Greg," Jack told me, "It's not how you accept winning. It's how you deal with losing that matters. Guys who can learn from losing are the ones who get ahead."

He said, "I never sat there on a green and said under my breath 'miss it' to one of my competitors. If they made it, good for them. They're doing something right, and now I have to be better. Maybe it's being better on the greens or walking the course or working on my swing, it doesn't matter. You say to the guy who beat you, 'You played well, you played better than I did.' And then you figure out how to win the next time."

I thought about that a lot over the years. Life isn't always as clear as golf. It's more complicated to figure out who wins and loses when you're talking about career and family instead of a game. I learned to pay attention to the people around me and figure out how to do better next time.

Barbara Nicklaus was a saint. It's easy to be nice to the other golfers, but she was nice to everyone—the fitness guys, the caddies, even the other players' wives. For example, the first gift my daughter got when she was born was a crystal bear with onyx eyes and nose and a diamond in it and a cashmere Teddy bear from Jack and Barbara. The card said it was from Jack and Barbara, but I know it was from Barbara. Jack didn't do that stuff. I mean, he was too busy. But Barbara was thoughtful like that. She was just revered by everybody.

As nice as Barbara was as a person, Fuzzy Zoeller was that funny. He had great talent and was one of the greatest ad-libbers I've ever met. He was a guy that said what he thought, but I never heard him say anything to hurt someone on purpose.

Fuzzy had a back problem that forced him to visit us in the van weekly. One day while getting treatment for his back problem, I told him, "Fuzzy you need to put some ice on your back tonight at the hotel."

He said, "If I have any ice left out of my cocktail, I will."

That same year at a tournament, I was standing on the platform outside the van with Fuzzy watching the patrons walk by and we noticed a very classy woman in a white pair of very tight pants. Fuzzy said, "Hey, Greg, do you like her?"

I said, "Yep, sure do."

I then thought he was going to the clubhouse after his treatment to get ready, but on his way I noticed he was talking to the woman in the white pants. A second later they turned toward the van, and he points to me. I wondered what he said to her because she had a big smile on her face.

Later that day when I saw Fuzzy, I asked him what he said to her.

"I said 'My friend in the van over there wants to have sex with you.'"

"Why did you say that?"

He said, "Because its true. You wanted her."

Fuzzy always told it like it was.

I said earlier that golf is unique in sports because the players pay their own way for tournaments, hire their own caddies, and buy their own tickets—as well as the tickets of anyone traveling with them. All of the guys had to hustle a lot for money. Payne Stewart, for instance, got paid $150,000 a year just to wear an Ebel watch back in the eighties, which wasn't a bad deal for him. But before that, Arnold Palmer had the longest running contract for sports equipment in the history of sports with Wilson golf clubs. And that contract wasn't really a contract, it was all on a handshake.

Of course, that's all changed. And Deane Beman is the guy that golfers need to give credit to for the game exploding. He was the commissioner of golf when the Tour exploded with TV money and sponsorships. Beman and his team are responsible for getting companies like AT&T, Buick, Coca-Cola, BellSouth, and so many others to sign on as sponsors.

Today, the tournament purses are enough to keep a golfer going, and that was due to the work that Beman and his team did. But I remember that Curtis Strange was the first golfer in history to win a million dollars in a year. Now that doesn't even get you in the top fifty.

The thing about Beman's work, though, is that he had to have a great product to sell to those sponsors. And that didn't happen without two people: Arnold Palmer and Jack Nicklaus.

Palmer got golf on TV. Or, to be a bit more accurate, he made golf on TV look good. Arnold was the ultimate golfer for the fans. And then Nicklaus came along, but he wasn't very well liked early in his career. They called him "Fat Jack" because he was a little overweight. The big problem was that he was beating Arnold Palmer's pants off. People didn't like that. Later in his career Jack got the respect of the fans, and then he was beloved. But Arnold from the day he got out there, everybody just loved that guy. Women wanted him, and men wanted to be like him. They wanted to dress like him. They wanted to play golf like him.

And there's a third guy who came along later who really pushed the money into the stratosphere: Tiger Woods. He brought a swagger and style and athleticism that golf hadn't seen before. Sure, some guys had some of that stuff in different proportions, but Tiger was the whole package, and he made the eyeballs—and the money—follow him everywhere.

I will say this, there is nobody today, other than Tiger, who even comes close to the accolades that Palmer and Nicklaus got. Nobody. Not in any sport. The only other sports figure that generated that kind of veneration, and maybe I'm a little bit biased, was Mickey Mantle. Willie Mays also had a lot of fans back then. And guys like Michael Jordan and LeBron James are pretty much household names, but the way the media followed those three guys around and generated hero-worship for them, that hasn't happened since Nicklaus and Palmer.

So I count it a blessing that I was able to meet so many of these figures, including Tiger. He's an icon—a legend already.

I met him when I was the medical director of the 2000 Tour championship in Atlanta. We couldn't bring in the trailers, so we had a locker room set up for us. One of the physical therapists I worked with said, "Hey, man, you want to go over and meet Tiger?"

I went over to meet Tiger, and we all went out for a beer afterwards. Couldn't have been nicer guy to hang out with. He can be a little standoffish with the media, and you have to understand that he'd been through a lot by then. It turned out that Tiger's the kind of guy that wants to go out and have a beer and have fun. It's a side to sports figures that not everyone gets to see.

We talked about his fitness book that he was working on and when I pushed for more, he said, with a big smile on his face, "It's top secret information, and if I told you I'd have to kill you." I was amazed at his physique. He reminded me of a football player, body-wise, not any golfer I had ever seen.

But I want to go back to talk about Arnold Palmer again. He was the king of the game that everyone loved; it was his star power that brought the game of golf to such popularity on TV. He was the first golfer to bring agents to the game. He is one of the people responsible for the modern success of the PGA Tour.

The times I was at Arnold's house in Orlando during the Tour stop, he was always fiddling with his clubs in his garage. He had twenty-five-gallon trashcans filled with hundreds of clubs. He was always changing grips and shafts, working on designs for Wilson and then his own brand.

Going Green: Life on the PGA Tour 1985-87

Fans would boo Jack Nicklaus back in the day when he would beat Arnold. Arnold was the most beloved golfer I ever knew. He was very nice to me, and he asked what the guys in the fitness trailer needed when we were at his tournament. I always said that Arnold would never quit playing while he physically could, and I absolutely expected him to die on a golf course.

Part of working for the PGA Tour was working for the LPGA and PGA Tour Champions as well. A Tour Champions event is where I met Palmer, and working that Tour also let me meet other golf legends, including Sam Snead.

Sam Snead was the winningest golfer in history, and I had the pleasure of treating him during the Senior Legends Team Championship at Onion Creek Country Club in Austin, TX. During the first day of the tournament, Bob Goalby, Sam's partner in the tournament, brought Sam into the fitness trailer. He introduced us, and I asked Sam how he hurt his back. Sam said that he had been dancing too much the night before. I laughed because Sam was in his 70s at the time, and I thought he was ribbing me. But Goalby confirmed that Sam was telling the truth.

I treated him the first day and also had the tournament doctor look at him. The doctor prescribed some anti-inflammatory medicine, and I told Sam I'd get his prescription filled and bring it to the hotel where he and I were staying.

When I got to his room, he invited me in, and there on the bed was a pretty, blond woman who looked to be around thirty just sitting there.

Sam turned to me, pointed to the woman, and said, "Sonny boy, that's how I really hurt my back last night." He called me that because he couldn't remember my name.

After treating Sam for the week, he came into the trailer and pulled out a crinkly, old-looking $20 bill, straightened it out on the edge of a table, and then reached in his back pocket and did the same with a five. He handed them to me and said, "Thanks, sonny boy."

Bob Goalby looked shocked, came over to me, and said, "You better frame that $25 because it's the only $25 that Sam ever gave to anyone."

Bob later told me about Sam's reputation for being the cheapest guy in golf history. I asked several of the older golfers on Tour about this reputation Sam had—all true. They told me that Sam used to say, "Watch your nickels and dimes, stay away from whisky, and never concede a putt."

Sam signed a golf glove and also gave me an old putter given to him by a fan that weekend and I still have those items today.

I was also a fan of several young stars of that era, and I was always happy to see them in the fitness trailer. I remember seeing Davis Love III a lot. He was one of the young Tour stars when I was on the Tour. I remember how long a hitter he was. At Atlanta Country Club during the BellSouth Open, he drove the 354-yard par 4 10th hole during an exhibition. He told me that he had learned that he needed to "back off" to control his game. He said he realized that hitting the ball farther was not best thing in his game. Davis was in the van all the time because of persistent back issues.

It turns out that Love's dad was a golfer instructor and would follow Davis during his golf career. We usually had strict rules about not letting anyone in but staff and golfers, but we relaxed the rules a bit for Davis Sr. He would get tired out on the course, and we'd let him come in and sit and chat. He was a great guy, and I felt like I lost a friend when he was killed in a plane crash in Hilton Head, SC.

If Davis Love III was in the trailer getting his back worked on, it was better than even odds that Fred Couples would be in there, too. They both had consistently bad backs, and Freddie would never listen to my advice on how to strengthen his back so that it wouldn't get injured.

Couples was one of the most charismatic golfers I met. Everybody liked him, but that didn't mean that everything was going great for him. Fred was also going through a not-so-good marriage, and the stress of that probably didn't help his back any.

If I saw Love and Couples a lot because of their back issues, then I saw Ben Crenshaw almost as much because of his videos. Ben was a true golf historian. I remember tapes of Bobby Jones teachings that he brought into the fitness van and played for us. He was also a true gentleman. He always had a smile and greeted you warmly. He was also a great host and helped me get a great deal on boots while in Austin during the Legends Tournament on the Senior PGA Tour stop. He also had a lot of theories about putting that he would never tire of sharing.

Crenshaw had his favorite topics of conversation, but Lee Trevino could talk about anything. Forever. He was the best talker I ever met in sports. I would tell people that Lee could talk to the wall for a half an hour—he never even needed a response. He visited the fitness trailer one day in Washington, DC, and asked for help with a stiff neck. He started talking and didn't let up for an hour. He didn't even stop to take a breath! Some of the other golfers didn't like Trevino because he talked constantly while playing, but he was one of the real great guys on and off the course.

Some of the guys didn't always bring the most reputable videotapes to the trailer. One time someone brought a stack of porn tapes which we all enjoyed until one guy ratted us out and had the commissioner, Deane Beman, call us. Sad to say that the tapes disappeared after that.

As I look over the list of golfers I met and admired, it's not hard to recognize that this was—and in many ways still is—a white man's game. And that's too bad. Any sport gets better when you have more people playing it. Better, smarter athletes show up, they challenge each other, and the game gets better. Look around at any sport and see if that isn't true.

I had the chance to meet and talk with Charlie Sifford, the first black golfer to play on the PGA Tour. I got to know him a little bit, and I asked him about what it was like. He said, "Greg, it was tough. I couldn't stay in the same hotels as other players. I couldn't eat at the same restaurants as other players."

I said, "Man, I don't get it."

"Greg," he said, "that was just the way it was back then. It was tough as a black man playing golf on the PGA Tour. I don't mean that to be derogatory toward anybody. It's just a fact."

That was not an easy conversation, but I'm glad I asked.

And there were a couple of other black players, like Jimmy Lee Thorpe, but there weren't many. Tiger certainly brought a lot of attention to that history, and now there are a few more black players, but not as many as I had hoped. Still I think there will be more, and the sport will be better because of it.

In fact, I believe that Tiger has done more for golf than almost any other player, along with Arnold Palmer. He brought golf to a whole new segment of the population and popularized golf all over the world as the most recognizable athlete since Muhammad Ali. Meeting Tiger was one of the thrills of my golf career because he was the greatest golfer I got to see in their prime. He hit shots that no other person on Tour could hit. He also had one of the two best minds on Tour: him and Raymond Floyd.

I loved the Tour, but golf was tough. We had to drive that truck. We would be six weeks on and a week off. We were there in the trailer from dawn to dusk and sometimes beyond. They could be really long days.

In those days, the season was a little different than today. We usually started on the West Coast at the Bob Hope Desert Classic in February. Then we'd have the West Coast swing, and that would take us from the Hope to LA to San Diego, which was the Andy Williams Open, which I called the Bing Crosby Clambake. Then they would tee up at Pebble Beach. The next stop was Hawaii, and we usually had a week off before that event. And that was always a great week because we would almost always head over to the islands before everyone else and get in a week of rest and relaxation.

It worked like this: United had a great deal for everyone because they were the official airlines for the PGA Tour. They would either give you a plane ticket home or a plane ticket to wherever you wanted to go. Whichever was cheaper. So what my fellow trainers and I would do is we'd fly to Hawaii for the first week off because the Hawaii ticket was always somehow cheaper than flying home. One of the guys, Mark Rawling, had a condo out there, so we'd spend a week playing golf, going to the beach, and doing all the touristy stuff. It was fabulous. The PGA Tour couldn't have treated employees better than the way they treated us. It was such a class organization. But we—the guys in the fitness trailer—were keeping the golfers healthy, which meant that the paying public was happy, and that meant that the PGA couldn't get the money to the bank fast enough.

It was great to be treated that well, but I also felt supremely lucky to work for that organization. I have a story that describes just how lucky I felt.

I was sitting next to Tom Watson in a bar in New Orleans on River Street. We were having a great time, drinking great beers, and eating great seafood, which I'm usually not a big fan of. We were just shooting the breeze, and I looked around and said, "You gotta be shitting me."

I was sitting there with Tom Watson, just like he's a buddy, which, you know, he was. He could be a little aloof, but he treated me great. And then I remembered how I met him.

It was my first golf tournament, the Bob Hope Desert Classic. Tom Kite came to the van and said to me—nobody else did this—he said, "Hey, You ever been to Palm Springs before?"

I said, "No."

"You want to go to dinner tonight?"

"Sure!"

He said, "Meet me at the Red Onion in Palm Springs."

So I met him there. We were sitting there enjoying dinner, and I looked over and saw Tom Watson. I had never seen him in person before. I looked at him and kept looking, until Kite said, "Okay, just tell me the truth. You want to meet Tom Watson, don't you?"

I said, "Would you mind?"

"Of course not!" So he waved, and Watson came right over. Turns out they were buddies.

Kite said, "Hey, I want you to meet Greg Johnson. He's going to be working on the fitness van."

Watson said, "Oh yeah, I heard about that."

He didn't come in a lot. He came in a few times, but he was just didn't have many physical problems at the time.

The fitness van never felt like a job. Sure, it was sometimes exhausting work, but it just felt like a gift from lady luck to be working there. How else could a guy like me hang out with guys like Kite and Watson?

I was happy that lady luck smiled on me like she did, but I learned a lot while working in sports. I learned important life lessons like how to deal with life when things don't go your way. Do you deal with the setback with grace and class and then get hungrier? Or do you sit and pout and cuss and scream and mutter under your breath at somebody, and blame it on somebody else? Jack Nicklaus told me to take personal responsibility for things that happen. And I saw that same attitude in many of the men and women I worked with over the years.

When I couldn't catch on with the major league outfit, I knew that I had to make a change. Was I frustrated and angry? Sure. And maybe some of it was political, but the only thing I could control was my reaction and my decision. I was sad to leave baseball. I loved my time with the sport. Did I know something even better was around the corner? No. I knew I had to keep moving, and I knew I didn't want to burn any bridges when I left. It's not easy to exit with grace and class, but people remember you for it. And the next chapter was better than I ever would have thought.

SEVEN

FAIRWAY DRIVE: PGA TOUR
PART 2, 1988-90

Those were the greatest five years of my life—bar none. The guys were so appreciative. Every year I'd get up a care package at Christmas from Jack Nicklaus. I'd guess that Jack had almost nothing to do with it. It was probably from Barbara, his wife, but it would be full of Golden Bear golf shirts, cashmere sweaters, golf balls, golf gloves, and such. Payne sent me stuff from Plus Four, which was his brand. Raymond Floyd sent stuff. The golfers just couldn't be nicer.

It's pretty obvious that you'd meet a lot of golfers while working on the PGA Tour. A lot of famous ones, and a lot of not-so-famous ones. I also knew from my days with the Braves, and my brief time with the USFL, that famous people like to hang around athletes. Olivia Newton-John was a great surprise when I was with the Braves. Maybe they played the game as a kid (probably not Olivia!), or, when it comes to golf, they were probably still playing it. Just nowhere near as well as the pros.

The players were usually pretty excited to meet the celebrities, too. A sort of mutual attraction happens among famous people. Who else are they going to get to complain to about crazy fans? And then there are the guys like me in the fitness trailer who get to hang around and meet both groups.

One of my biggest thrills during my golf career was to meet my favorite actor, Clint Eastwood, at Pebble Beach. Eastwood was in the Pro Am portion of the tournament paired with Raymond Floyd. I asked Floyd weeks before the tournament to please bring Eastwood into the fitness van for all of us to meet him.

During the tournament, we were in the van watching our usual set of movies, and that day we had Dirty Harry on the big screen. My back was to the door of the trailer when I heard a familiar voice say, "Hello, boys. How do you like the movie?"

I turned quickly and there, in real life, were Clint Eastwood and Raymond Floyd. I was so glad Raymond hadn't let me down. Clint was just as I thought he'd be—and better. He wasn't dressed like someone with tons of money, just like in his movies; he spoke softly, but firmly. He stayed in the van visiting for over an hour and was so classy. He signed an autograph to me and also gave me a card with a special note to the manager of the Hog's Breath Inn, his restaurant. When I showed up, I was treated like a king and never paid for food or drinks that first time—or for years later.

Sammy Davis was the name sponsor for the Great Hartford Open in Connecticut. Sammy was always there to greet the players and Tour officials when we arrived. When I first met

Sammy in the lockerroom, he said hello and immediately asked me if this was the first time I'd met a black Jew. He always wore tons of gold around his neck and on his wrist. But his love for gold showed up pretty much everywhere, even his golf clubs were gold-plated.

Some of these meetings were pretty ephemeral. I had an encounter with former President Ford at the Bob Hope Desert Classic that didn't result in a conversation, but I'll never forget it. Mr. Ford was playing in the Pro Am, though I hadn't seen him around the course. I was driving a golf cart to the clubhouse, and, as I was going around the corner of a golf path, I came up on a couple of people and nearly missed hitting one, who turned out to be President Ford. The look on his face was not a happy one, and the Secret Service agent certainly didn't have a smile on his face, either.

I was a bit closer, and not a threat, the next time I met a President—or a soon-to-be President. I was invited to eat at the White House in 1988 by a friend of one of the golfers, Bob Eastwood, who had arranged for a couple of PGA Tour officials and a few others of us to go to dinner there. Back then, the security wasn't as strict, but the Secret Service called my relatives to verify my place of birth, schooling, and such details. The meal was awesome; we ate on the new China that had just been purchased by Mrs. Reagan. The Secret Service did the security screening because our dinner also included a private tour of the entire White House. We went everywhere except the private living quarters of then-President Ronald Reagan. One of my favorite places was the basement. We saw lots of furniture that previous Presidents had used, some old paintings, and passageways that led off to parts unknown.

As we were walking through the hall near the Situation Room, out walked Vice President Bush. He didn't say anything, but I did get a smile and a nod of the head. I left with lots of memories and a book of matches with a gold-embossed logo of the Presidency, which I still have.

Presidents—either at the White House or not—seem to really like golf. But they aren't the only politicians that like the game as much as I do. And they come from both sides of the political aisle.

The week before the 1988 Hawaiian Open tournament, I was in Hawaii with Gene Lane and Paul Callaway. We were in a condo that Gary Koch, a Tour player, had given to us to use before the tournament. While the guys went to the beach, I decided to get in eighteen holes (I'm telling you, I really do love this game!). I was playing the hole on the Ocean course called "The Little Grand Canyon," but a threesome ahead was slowing me down. When I reached the green I was asked if I wanted to join them. It took me just a second to recognize the person who was asking, Tip O'Neil. He had a unique, deep, firm voice. He was very nice to talk with and was a golf lover. When he asked what I did and I told him, he was inquisitive about my job. But the first thing I noticed about his game was that his size—he was big around his waist—didn't help his golf game. His girth meant that his swing was not very good, but he still hit it fairly straight. We finished that nine, and I headed back to the clubhouse.

Working for the PGA Tour also gave me the opportunity to work for some LPGA Tour events. I would have been glad to work more, but the Tour schedule and geography didn't line up all that often. Those women were all amazing athletes, and a few of them really made an impression.

My favorite golfer from the LPGA was Dottie Pepper. She was a super person, and I enjoyed her company while treating her for some back issues. She was a very attractive woman, and I can admit pretty openly that I had a little crush on her. We had dinner a couple of times after treatment, and I was happy to be seen escorting her around the restaurant.

A couple of golfers have made a huge impact both in the US and in Asia. A lot of people know Tiger Woods, of course, but Se-ri Pak was one of the greatest golfers of all time and a legend in Korea. She came into the van at the tournament in Atlanta, the 1993 Chick-fil-A Classic, with some wrist problems. As beautiful as she was, she was even nicer as a person. We did not speak much, but she certainly was one of my favorite female golfers.

Nancy Lopez was one of the classiest golfers on the LPGA Tour, and one of the greats—she was inducted into the World Golf Hall of Fame in 1987. She wasn't just a player, though, she also hosted the Chick-fil-A Tournament in Atlanta. She was always very friendly and kind. Every year, she would come by the trailer and ask if we needed anything, then she would thank us for working with the tournament and for helping the golfers participating.

Lopez and I had a connection that was a little more special than most because her husband, Ray Knight, was a Major

League Baseball player with the Cincinnati Reds. He played in the big leagues while I was with the Braves, so we always had a lot to talk about.

Another famous woman I met during an LPGA event wasn't a golfer. I met Martina Navratilova at the Hilton Head Tournament in 1989. She had just finished playing the Hilton Head tennis tournament when she came into the trailer, which had just arrived from the Masters.

I was in the trailer when I heard a knock on the door. I opened it, and there stood Martina. She introduced herself, and I said, "I know who you are!" I knew I was talking with the greatest female tennis player in history.

She smiled and said that her wrist was bothering her and was wondering if I would take a look.

During the hour she was in the van, I was pleasantly surprised by how nice she was and how willing she was to talk with me. I was really impressed with how fit she was. She had the most chiseled body I had ever seen on a woman. While she getting her TENS (Transcutaneous Electrical Nerve Stimulation) treatment, there was another knock on the door. This time it was a different beautiful woman. She introduced herself as Cindy Nelson, Martina's girlfriend.

Cindy came in and asked Martina, "How's your wrist?"

While the treatment continued, Cindy was also very pleasant and asked about my job and how much I liked working on Tour. When the two left the van, Martina caught me checking out Cindy as they walked away. Without saying a word, Martina reached around Cindy's waist and grabbed her ass.

Then she caught me eye, and I just smiled as they walked out of sight.

I expect that Martina stayed around for some of the golf tournament that followed her tennis competition. Most athletes are fans of other sports, which makes sense. A lot of them grew up playing a bunch of different sports until they found the one they really excelled at. But my favorite crossover story brings golf and football together.

I had only spent a couple of months with the USFL, but my friendship with Archie Griffin was, I thought, pretty solid. So when I was going through some phone numbers, shooting the shit with some golfers in the fitness truck, and I landed on Archie's number. It was the Memorial Tournament in Dublin, OH, and I said, "You know, I'm in Ohio. I'm going to call him."

One of guys, Bob Eastwood, looked up and said, "You don't know Archie Griffin."

"Wanna bet?" I said, "I'll bet you 20 bucks."

He said, "Yeah, I'll bet you 20 bucks you don't know Archie."

I smiled, "Watch me."

I dialed the number and Archie answered the phone. I put him on speaker and said, "Hey, Arch, this is Greg Johnson."

Without missing a beat, he said, "Greg! How're you doing, man? What are you up to these days?"

I said, "I'm working on the PGA Tour. The Memorial is in Dublin this weekend."

"Oh yeah, that's right," he said. "I heard about that. Buncha the guys are interested in that tournament."

"You planning to come out?"

"Yeah, man. I'd like to, but I didn't get anything set up."

I said, "Well, I'll get you some tickets."

"That'd be great!"

He showed up, but I only saw him for a few minutes. He's Archie Griffin, after all, and a legend. Especially in Ohio. And Eastwood paid up.

It's sort of funny that Eastwood made that bet. I had my book of phone numbers right there in front of him, so why did he think I didn't have a connection to Archie Griffin? But sports isn't always about being smart. A lot of times, it isn't. It's true that these men and women had physical gifts beyond what any of us have, and they can think about their bodies and how they move around better than most of us. I used to say, "There's a two-cent brain operating a million-dollar golf swing." Those golfers could do amazing things with a club and ball, but they couldn't think their way through the course.

It's like that movie, Tin Cup. Kevin Costner's character is leading going into the final holes, but he gets distracted by thinking he should make a shot that he can't—at least, he can't on that day. So he loses. Not because he can't hit the ball great but because he's not thinking about how to play the course. The brain is more powerful than the body. A lot of pro golfers with great smarts and just decent skills have solid careers.

Jack Nicklaus was one of the smart guys (as well as being a great athlete), and, as I mentioned, I followed his advice to step away from the Tour and settle in one place with my family. That conversation happened at the 1989 Shell Houston

Open in Houston. I told him that I had just learned that I was going to be a dad.

"You're going to quit, aren't you?" Nicklaus asked, "You got to."

I looked at him for a minute, "You're kidding me, right, Jack?"

"Let me tell you a little story," he said, "When I started playing golf, I had to. I had to play golf and do other things to make a living, to put food on the table. Golf was not a multimillion-dollar business when I started."

"I wasn't around very much to be part of Steve and Jackie's life as young kids," he went on, referring to his two oldest boys. "And Barbara, if it wasn't for her, those kids wouldn't have grown up how they grew up. Now I can give them big positions in my company, and I can give them all the money, but I can't make up for those times that I wasn't there as a dad."

"Greg," he said, "do yourself a favor and your kid a favor, too: get a real job, be at home, be part of raising your kid so that they can grow up to be a positive influence in society as an adult. You'll thank yourself for it."

And I said, "Yeah..." To be honest, I kind of blew it off at first, but it stayed with me. After a little while, I talked to my wife about the idea. Six weeks later, I quit.

Leaving the PGA Tour was one of the hardest decisions I ever made. In my entire professional career, I had never done anything so rewarding. The people I worked with were great—the golfers as well as my colleagues in the fitness

trailer all the way up to the commissioner. The whole opera-
tion was classy and fun.

But one thing I really miss that not a lot of people talk
about—and I know this will sound a little greedy, but it's
true—is the schwag. We all got sets of clubs and great clothes
for free. We got cashmere sweaters and FootJoy shoes. The
sponsors sent shirts, pants, hats, gloves—everything but
underwear. I have gloves in my closet that I haven't opened
yet, and that was thirty years ago! I couldn't wear all of it, so I
used to take half the stuff and send it to my younger brother
who was still in college.

So it was tough to walk away from the PGA. But I kept
thinking back to something else Jack said to me when he
talked about figuring out how to win—how to do better—the
next time.

I had learned a lot over the years from taking that advice
to heart. And I knew I had to do better. Maybe not a better
job—nothing will beat the PGA—but better as a family man
and medical professional. I knew I could help my family and
other people, and that's what I went on to do.

One of the things I did in the mid-1990s was publish a
couple of articles for amateur golfers who wanted to feel
better and to play better golf. I worked with Dr. James L.
Chappius, an orthopedic spine surgeon in Atlanta. We published "Super Six Stretching Exercises for Golf" and "Super
Six Strengthening Exercises for Golf" in Physician and Sports
Medicine, a prestigious medical journal specific to my field.

I said earlier that it's important not to burn bridges. When
you walk away from a job—whether you love it or not—you

want to leave on the best possible terms. That was definitely the case with the PGA because, even though I left the Tour in 1990, I was asked in 1994 to become the medical director of a golf tournament in Winder, GA, the Gene Sarazen World Open.

The tournament honored not only one of the greatest golfers in history, but a person who all golfers revered.

In order to get an invitation, you had to have won an open championship somewhere in the world—or get a special invitation from Gene Sarazen personally. Golfers like Payne Stewart and Jack Nicklaus were regulars at the tournament, and everyone who got a personal invitation accepted because of the respect Sarazen commanded.

I was the medical director for this tournament for the five years it was in Georgia. I was grateful for the opportunity and had a lot of fun. Not only did I get the chance to work on the PGA Tour again but I was also able to to do so near my home in Atlanta. It may have been the highlight of my sports medicine career—after the full-time sports jobs—to work the Sarazen. Every year at the tournament we had a friendly, relaxed atmosphere, and I had a chance to reconnect with old friends. Like my time on the Tour, I have a lot of great memories from that tournament.

My fondest memory of the tournament was having Jack Nicklaus and Payne there to talk about our friendships. I also remember meeting John Daly for the first time. I was in the treatment room with Fuzzy Zoeller. He saw Daly walk by and called out to him. Fuzzy asked if I had ever met Daly, and I said no. When I shook his hand, Daly responded by saying,

"Where can I take a shit around here?" Not the first guy to ask me that, but definitely the first guy not to say, "It's nice to meet you" first.

My favorite winner was Frank Nobilo. I treated him during both his wins at the Sarazen. He was just a great guy, and I really enjoyed working with him.

My personal favorite detail is that Gene Sarazen had a great golf cart that was made especially for him because of the particular needs he had as a grand old man of golf. The tournament was held in November, which is a cold part of the year even in Atlanta, so the organizers had a cart made with sides and a heater to keep the ninety-four-year-old legend nice and warm. He looked great zipping around the course in his heated cart.

A more complicated memory that stands out to me involves Payne Stewart, a good friend and one of Sarazen's favorite golfers. I was at the driving range with Payne, and I was clearly struggling with something. Payne asked me if I was happy in my married life. I asked him why he would ask that question. He said he could tell that something wasn't quite right with me.

"You got me," I told him. "I'm not doing great."

Payne quickly said, "Listen, Greg, I've gotten right with God, my wife, and my family. I have twenty million dollars in the bank, and I'm going to use my money to spend more time with my family. That's what's important." He looked at me and continued, "Either get right with your wife and fix it or get out."

Fairway Drive: PGA Tour Part 2, 1988-90

A few months later the tournament announced that it would no longer continue. Right about that time I had a nightmare, though it had nothing to do with golf. In the nightmare, I kept hearing "fix it or get out." It woke me up, and I sat there in the dark for a minute, then woke up my wife and said, "We are done." I was divorced six months later. When Payne was killed in a plane crash, it was one of the saddest days of my life. Payne was a true friend and every time the US Open is on, I think of him.

Of course, Gene Sarazen wasn't the only golfer to keep playing late into his life, though ninety-four is longer than most. Golfing is a sport you can play for a long time, and the PGA Tour figured out that some of the most popular golfers could still play a great game and people were still willing to watch. So the PGA Tour Champions was born, though it's been through a couple of name changes before they settled on that one. Golf is one of the few sports where you could do that. You're not going to see a senior baseball league or senior NFL. The older golfers can't drive like the young ones, but they still have a good control game and work the short game well.

What really made the Champions succeed though was getting Jack Nicklaus and Arnold Palmer to sign on. Those two guys were always at the front of the media pack, so it's no surprise that they made that Tour a success as well.

But those weeks with the Sarazen always ended with me going back to my real-world job. Each year was bittersweet, but the first year away from full-time professional sports was hard. It was a difficult transition for a professional who had enough degrees and experience built up to have great opportunities back in the real world. But my transition was easy compared to some of the ballplayers I knew. A lot of people don't understand how hard it is for ballplayers who play through three, four, five years, and get to the end of their career. They're in their twenties, which is really young, and they suddenly have to find something else to do after that. They've played baseball or golf or football or whatever all their life, and they're used to being the center of attention wherever they go. And then they have to get a nine-to-fiver like everyone else. They join the rest of us, nobody pays them a lot of attention any more, and the real world uses different skills than what they've been training for their whole lives.

For some of these kids sports was all they could do. A lot of them didn't finish college. Some of these kids get started really young—sixteen, seventeen years old. More than a few aren't from the US, either. They come from the Dominican Republic, Mexico, and places even farther away. They have these physical gifts, but there's nothing set up to help these kids when their careers end. They just have to go figure it out.

The money for journeyman players is pretty good, and for young people who have money for the first time in their life, it's a huge temptation to get all the nice things they've ever wanted. But when they get cut they have to figure out what to do with what they have left, which a lot of times isn't much. And they have to ask what they're going to do for the rest of their life. It's a scary place to be in.

I was in a different situation. I had a master's degree, and I was able to integrate myself into sports medicine at the community level. I started working in a sports medicine clinic covering a high school in Taylors, South Carolina. I had seen the evolution and growth of sports medicine, and now it was available for high school kids, and it was a lot better than what I had to work with back when I was their age. It felt good to be working in the community and spending time with my daughter, watching her grow up. I missed the close connection to sports, but it still felt like I had made the right decision. And then a couple years later I had a conversation that confirmed my belief that I had made the right choice.

I had a secretary, Linda, who had worked for me in a physical therapy facility in Atlanta where I was the director. We had both both moved on to other things, but we ran into each other again after several years. I asked how she was doing and what she was doing for work. She said that she had become a nanny. I asked her if she liked it, and she said, "Y'know it's really sad."

That surprised me. "What do mean?"

"This family I'm working for," Linda said, "they're super successful. They each make in the mid-six figures. They have everything. But they never spend any time with their kids—a girl and boy who are just great kids. Even on the weekends, the parents say they have things to do and errands to run, so they call me and ask if I can come over. And I do."

I didn't really know what to say, but she kept talking.

"And here's the saddest part," she said. "The kids came up to me one day and said, 'We love you more than our parents.'"

And that made me think, as a parent, about how crushingly heartbreaking that would be if my daughter said that to me. So I knew right then and there that I had made the right decision all those years ago. Jack Nicklaus was right. We're not here to be successful. We're not here to have our name in lights. We're not here to make a lot of money. We're not here for our own self-gratification. If we're lucky enough to become a parent, then the best thing we'll ever do in our life is to raise a good kid to become a contributing adult.

I don't know what happened to Linda and those kids, but I was damned glad I had made the right choice.

AFTERWORD

When I was in high school, my parents were told I wasn't college material. Like a lot of teens I was immature and didn't know what I wanted to do, and it was easy to drift, which meant not paying attention in school. But sports gave me the impetus to make good grades because if I didn't, I couldn't stay on the team. I had to make the grades, or I was gone.

So sports kept me in school. To do the thing that I loved, sports, I had to keep working at something I didn't love so much, school. So sports were a great reinforcement to stay in school and get the grades.

But the thing is, I got into a habit of learning. It became so much a part of me that I now believe that if you're not learning, you're dying. I always try to learn three things that I didn't know yesterday. It keeps me alive. I also try to keep in mind that tomorrow is promised to no one, as the old saying goes. So I try to keep learning as part of making each day count.

Now, that lesson is more clear than ever. I've got four stents in my coronary arteries right now. When I had that done almost five years ago, I had no real symptoms. I had gone in for a routine stress test, and they decided that they needed to do a nuclear stress test, which is where they take an image of your heart while you're working out or after you work out. They didn't like what they saw, so they scheduled me for a procedure where they put a catheter in your wrist and run a wire up to your heart. You're awake for all of it, which feels really weird, and I watched it on a bank of screens they had set up. Which was also really weird.

"Huh," the doctor said, "this doesn't look good."

"Man," I said, "I don't want to hear that. Just give me some more meds, and it'll be fine."

Of course, that's not what they did.

After the stents were in, the doctor came into my room to talk about the procedure.

"How'd it go?" I said.

"It went great," he said. Then added, "You're lucky you didn't come in here in a body bag."

He took a deep breath, "Have you ever heard of a widowmaker?"

"Like a wild pitch?"

He laughed, "No, a widowmaker is when one of the arteries around your heart balloons out, and if it bursts, you're going to die in two minutes. That's what you had."

When you have things like that happen, you have a different perspective on life. It makes you think about what's really important. So you want to keep learning, and you want to reflect a little more on what life has given you. These lessons feel all the more important to me now. As I was finishing this book, I found out that I'm going to be a grandfather. My first grandchild! And sure, I'll want to be like my grandfather was for me and help them experience the, well, wide world of sports. More than that, though, I want to make sure that I pass on these lessons. I want to help this new child become the best adult they can be.

For me, I've been given some great opportunities and lessons through sports. It's taught me how to be humble. I learned humility by realizing how lucky I am. I wasn't the best person for all these jobs. I was in the right place at the right time. And luck goes a long way in life, you know? I mean, you still have to do the work. You still need to want to make something of yourself. But even as small a thing as having good people around you in life means you have some luck.

Here's a story that really gets to the question of luck.

I was applying for a job at Health South in the mid 90s. I was doing pretty well with the process, and I had an interview set up with their VP. I walked into his office, and he said, "You know, Greg, I had to meet you."

"Why's that?"

"Even if I don't hire you, I had to meet you. I have never met anybody who had Frank Jobe, Jimmy Andrews, Hank Aaron, AND Jack Nicklaus listed as references. And I want to find out, is this right? Is this the truth?"

I said, "Go ask Dr. Andrews."

He sat there and looked at for a moment, then slapped his hand down on his desk.

"Alright, man," he said. "We want you on our team."

All of my experience in sports gave me an opportunity that would last the rest of my career because sports set me up to work for the biggest healthcare company in the world.

I also learned that it's not what you take in life that gives life meaning. It's what you give. It's important to remember that. You should give back if you've been blessed enough. Jack Nicklaus said this to me more than once, "If you're blessed enough to get nice things in life, give it back to somebody." Whenever he said that, it always reminded me of a time when I was a young man.

The first love of my life was a Puerto Rican girl. I was 19 years old. We had been dating for a while, and then one day her father didn't come home from work. He just left them. We learned later that he had gone back to Puerto Rico, and they never saw him back in the States again. He left three girls and two boys for his wife to take care of, and I never understood it. But one of the boys was an athlete, and I kind of took him on as a younger brother because he didn't have a father figure or a big brother figure. He was a pretty good athlete, and I taught him how to play golf, taught him to play baseball. I've kept track of him, and he's done pretty well for himself.

Maybe he'd be ok without my showing up, but I know that's part of what got me where I am. I didn't know that at the time, of course. I was just a kid myself, really. But giving back to others, that's important. It's also important to remember that we don't get where we're going without some help from others. Remembering that help keeps you humble, and it makes it easier to pass that help on to others. And sports made it easy for me to pass that help on.

Another important lesson I learned, and that I've mentioned a few times already, was that you don't ever burn a bridge. I think that's something that everybody thinks they need to do or they want to do: burn bridges. They walk out of a situation that they think wasn't good, and that's just a natural impulse—you throw a match and the whole thing burns as you walk away. When the words are out, they're out, and you can't take them back. But the thing is, you never know when you might need to cross back over again.

For my career, the sports world and the medical world are small entities. Everybody knows everybody, it's not even six degrees of separation. It's like one or two. I think a lot of professions are like that. So if you have to leave, try to leave on the best possible terms.

My career didn't end when I left the golf tour. I still had thirty more years to go, and I've been blessed.

Shortly after leaving sports, a guy gave me a shot at running a physical therapy practice, which was great, except that I'm not a physical therapist. But I did it. A few years later, I moved on to run an orthopedic practice with a staff of over a hundred.

I had those opportunities because of sports. Because I met and worked with men like Jim Andrews, Don Fauls, and Frank Jobe. I got lucky, I know, but I worked hard for that luck, I never stopped learning, and I never burned bridges behind me.

Sports has given me so much in my life. I've been able to make a living, meet some great people, travel all over the world, learn a lot about life, and suffer personal heartbreaks before coming back as a better person because of sports.

I found a way to stay out of trouble as a youth, I stayed away from drugs and underage drinking, and I was able to meet the people who have made me who I am today.

But the most important lesson I learned was how to work together with others. To wrap it up, I'd like to add something that Bob Hope once said in a song, "Thanks for the memories!"

GREATEST HITS

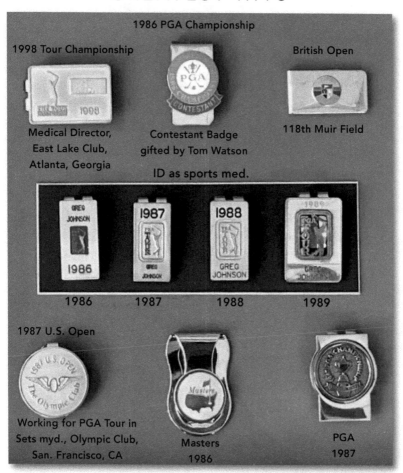

1986 PGA Championship

1998 Tour Championship

British Open

Medical Director,
East Lake Club,
Atlanta, Georgia

Contestant Badge
gifted by Tom Watson
ID as sports med.

118th Muir Field

1986

1987

1988

1989

1987 U.S. Open

Working for PGA Tour in
Sets myd., Olympic Club,
San. Francisco, CA

Masters
1986

PGA
1987

When you're in the sports business, you see a lot of play-ers and a lot of stadiums. Many of us who spent time in the business have our favorites, and I'm no different. Reader, if you and I ever have a chance to sit down with a beer, I'd be happy to argue with you about all of the statements I'm going to make in the next few pages!

Favorite NCAA Football Field

This is an easy choice, Doak Campbell Stadium, home of the 'Noles.

Best NCAA Football Fans

I know you're expecting me to say Florida State fans, and they had a special standing in my all-time lists. But I think the best fans are those who pull for the Nebraska Cornhuskers. When we went to Lincoln, NE, to play the top-ten-ranked Cornhuskers their fans were fabulous—even after we won the game. When the final whistle blew, the fans stood up and gave us a standing ovation. Absolutely great fans!

Favorite Major League Baseball Stadium

There is no doubt in my mind about this one: Dodger Stadium in Los Angeles. The weather is perfect, the field is beautiful, and the city isn't bad, either. The flip side of the coin for me was Olympic Stadium in Montreal. Built for the 1976 Olympic Games, the place was falling apart by 1981. I felt bad for that city.

Favorite Pro Football Field

Lambeau Field, Green Bay, WI. I go back a long way with that stadium. It may not be the most cutting edge in terms of technology and entertainment away from the field, but it will always be my favorite.

Best Golf Course I Ever Played

Spyglass in Pebble Beach, CA. The views are spectacular and the weather is (almost always) great.

Best Group of Golf Courses in One Place

A single golf course can be great, but what if you want to just go to one place and hit a lot of great links? I have your destination mapped out for you, but my answer probably will surprise most golfers: Westchester County, NY. Within five miles, a golfer can find Westchester Country Club, Old Oaks, and Winged Foot. These are all old-style courses that can be hard to find these days.

Favorite Sport

This answer might also be a surprise, given all my love for golf. But my favorite sport is college football. It gave me my start in sports, and it's still my favorite thing to watch. The fans are so dedicated to their teams and schools, and it has a much different atmosphere than professional football. My favorite team won't be a surprise: Florida State.

Favorite Pro Sport

National Football League. I guess the lesson here is that I'd rather play golf but watch football.

Favorite NFL Team

The Green Bay Packers. I was born in Wisconsin, and I have been a Packer Backer since the early 1960s. My grandfather brought me all kinds of Packer goodies when he came to visit, and I've always considered myself a cheese head, even though I only lived there for a few years after I was born. I guess the Florida teams just never replaced my Packers.

Favorite Baseball Player

Mickey Mantle. Sometimes, you just can't shake the influences from when you're a kid. Mantle was always larger than life and I became an instant fan when I first saw him in the early 60s.

Favorite Moment in Sports

Given that he was my favorite baseball player, my favorite moment in sports was when I got to meet Mickey Mantle in Charleston, SC.

Best Pitcher I Ever Saw

I saw a lot of great pitchers while I worked for the Braves, but I will always believe that Nolan Ryan was the best. He was known for his 100-mile-an-hour fastball, but he had great control—and a mean breaking ball as well.

Favorite Teammate

Dale Murphy. He was just a great human being. He was the consummate ball player and a generous person. I never heard him say anything bad about anyone. He played hard, treated everyone with respect, and he was never bigger than the game or the people around him.

Toughest Fans in Major League Baseball

Philadelphia. Those fans were tough. They expected great baseball, and, when they didn't get it, they let their team know. But they were tough on all the teams. They even booed Santa Claus at an Eagles game.

Best People I've Ever Met

When someone asks about the best person I've ever met, I can't narrow it down to one. For me, there are three people who I think are truly great human beings who make the people around them better. They are: Bobby Bowden, former head football coach at Florida State; Dale Murphy, baseball play and teammate with the Braves; and Archie Griffin, football player with the Jacksonville Bulls of the USFL. They treated everybody with respect. They had great morals. They were intelligent. Those three people are the best human beings I've ever met in my life.

Best Job

I know I've mentioned this a few times, but it has to be said again. My best job ever was as an athletic trainer on the PGA Tour. I loved the game even before I got a job in it, and I grew up idolizing Tom Watson and Arnold Palmer. Then I not only got to meet them, but I got the chance to get to know them as friends. Yep. Best job ever.

Speechless Moments

Even with meeting lots of famous people, I had two entirely speechless moments. The first was when I met Mickey Mantle. The second was when I met Halle Berry.

Mickey Mantle was my idol and I was just stunned to meet him and then hang out over dinner and beers. When I met Halle, she had just had been voted the most beautiful woman in the world. She was at a dinner for the Braves, and her husband at the time, David Justice, introduced us. I could hardly get the word "hello" out of my mouth, but she was gracious and friendly.

Most Influential People in My Life

I've had a lot to say about sports figures, but I want talk about other people, too.

My Grandfather, Ray C. Johnson, and my mother [Jan; she was always there to take me to events, pick me up after school and practice]. My grandfather introduced me to sports at an early age, and that exposure set me on course for life. My mother is the happiest person I've ever known. She loves life, people, and her family. I don't know anyone that doesn't like her. To this day, she teaches me what a person should be and how to love life every day to its fullest. I'm sure glad my daughter Chelsea takes after her grandmother.

Most Important Person I Met in Life

Amy Newmark, my wife. She has put up with so much from me that I can't believe she still wants to hang around. She is also generous, loving, and present for all her friends and family. Family is so important to her, and she is the love of my life.

Favorite Moment in Life

The best thing that happened to me was when my daughter Chelsea was born. We are not put on this earth to make a lot of money, to be successful, or to get our name on a building. But if we are lucky enough to have children, our job is to raise children to be good human beings who contribute positively to the world they live in. I got that advice from Jack Nicklaus, and I follow that advice to this day. I did my best with her, but I believe I got lucky with a great kid. My daughter was never trouble, never got into trouble, stayed away from drugs, made good grades, and has gone on to start a family of her own. I am now and will always be proud of her.

And now I'm even more proud because she's made me a grandfather in 2021 to beautiful baby boy Alexander Dantuma. I can't express how much joy that brings to me—and I'm feeling blessed to share that joy with you.

CPSIA information can be obtained
at www.ICGtesting.com
Printed in the USA
LVHW081508051021
699577LV00016B/695